Praise for *The Pandemic Century*

A *FINANCIAL TIMES* BEST HEALTH BOOK OF 2019
A *NEW YORK TIMES* BOOK *REVIEW* EDITORS' CHOICE

"Gripping."
—Barbara Kiser, *Nature*

"[A] riveting, vivid history of modern disease outbreaks. . . . A fascinating account of a deeply important topic—for if the past 100 years have taught us anything, it is that new diseases and viral strains will inevitably beset us, no matter how sophisticated science becomes."
—Robin McKie, *Observer*

"A lively but less than reassuring read for those on exotic travels."
—Anjana Ahuja, *Financial Times*

"Infectious diseases remain among the most urgent health threats we face, but too often are considered something that happens to other people, far away. In our interconnected world, this is no longer true, as Mark Honigsbaum shows. His unique account drives home the human impact of epidemics, and the need for increased preparedness."
—Jeremy Farrar, director of the Wellcome Trust

THE
PANDEMIC
CENTURY

ALSO BY MARK HONIGSBAUM

A History of the Great Influenza Pandemics:
Death, Panic and Hysteria, 1830–1920

Living with Enza:
The Forgotten Story of Britain and the Great Flu Pandemic of 1918

The Fever Trail:
In Search of the Cure for Malaria

Valverde's Gold:
In Search of the Last Great Inca Treasure

THE
PANDEMIC
CENTURY

ONE HUNDRED YEARS OF

PANIC, HYSTERIA,

AND HUBRIS

MARK HONIGSBAUM

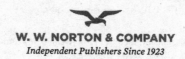

W. W. NORTON & COMPANY
Independent Publishers Since 1923

For information about permission to reproduce selections from this book, write to
Permissions, W. W. Norton & Company, Inc., 500 Fifth Avenue, New York, NY 10110

For information about special discounts for bulk purchases, please contact
W. W. Norton Special Sales at specialsales@wwnorton.com or 800-233-4830

Manufacturing by LSC Communications, Harrisonburg
Book design by Chris Welch
Production manager: Anna Oler

The Library of Congress has cataloged a previous edition of this book as follows:

Names: Honigsbaum, Mark, author.
Title: The pandemic century : one hundred years of panic, hysteria, and hubris /
Mark Honigsbaum.
Description: First edition. | New York : W. W. Norton & Company, [2019] |
Includes bibliographical references and index.
Identifiers: LCCN 2018048424 | ISBN 9780393254754 (hardcover)
Subjects: | MESH: Pandemics—history | History, 20th Century | History, 21st Century
Classification: LCC RA650.5 | NLM WA 11.1 | DDC 614.4/90904—dc23
LC record available at https://lccn.loc.gov/2018048424

ISBN 978-0-393-54131-1 pbk.

W. W. Norton & Company, Inc., 500 Fifth Avenue, New York, N.Y. 10110
www.wwnorton.com

W. W. Norton & Company Ltd., 15 Carlisle Street, London W1D 3BS

1 2 3 4 5 6 7 8 9 0

FOR MARY-LEE

"Everybody knows that pestilences have a way of recurring in the world; yet somehow we find it hard to believe in ones that crash down on our heads from a blue sky. There have been as many plagues as wars in history; yet plagues and wars always take people by surprise."

—ALBERT CAMUS, *The Plague*

CONTENTS

THE
PANDEMIC
CENTURY

SHARKS AND OTHER PREDATORS

Sharks never attack bathers in the temperate waters of the North Atlantic. Nor can a shark sever a swimmer's leg with a single bite. That's what most shark experts thought in the blisteringly hot summer of 1916 as New Yorkers and Philadelphians flocked to the beaches of northern New Jersey in search of relief from the sweltering inland temperatures. That same summer the East Coast had been gripped by a polio epidemic, leading to the posting of warnings about the risk of catching "infantile paralysis" at municipal pools. The Jersey shore was considered a predator-free zone, however.

"The danger of being attacked by a shark," declared Frederic Lucas, director of the American Museum of Natural History in July 1916, "is infinitely less than that of being struck by lightning and . . . there is practically *no* danger of an attack from a shark about our coasts." As proof, Lucas pointed to the reward of $500 that had been offered by the millionaire banker Hermann Oerlichs "for an authenticated case of a man having being attacked by a shark in temperate waters [in the United States, north of Cape Hatteras, North Carolina]"—a sum that had gone unclaimed since Oerlichs had posted the challenge in the *New York Sun* in 1891.

But Oerlichs and Lucas were wrong, and so were Dr. Henry Fowler and Dr. Henry Skinner, the curators of Philadelphia's Academy of Natural Science who had categorically stated, also in 1916, that a shark lacked the power to sever a man's leg. The first exception to these *known* facts had come on the evening of July 1, 1916, when Charles Epting Vansant, a wealthy young broker holidaying in New Jersey with his wife and family, decided to go for a predinner swim near his hotel at Beach Haven. A graduate of the University of Pennsylvania's class of 1914, Vansant, or "Van" to his chums, was a scion of one of the oldest families in the country—Dutch immigrants who had settled in the United States in 1647—and famed for his athleticism. If he had any concerns about entering the cool Atlantic waters that evening, they would have been offset by the familiar sight of the beach lifeguard, Alexander Ott, a member of the American Olympic swimming team, and a friendly Chesapeake Bay retriever that ran up to him as he slid into the surf. In the fashion of young Edwardian men of the time, Vansant swam straight out beyond the lifelines, before turning to tread water and call to the dog. By now his father, Dr. Vansant, and his sister, Louise, had arrived on the beach and were admiring his form from the lifeguard station. Much to their amusement, the hound refused to follow. Moments later, the reason became apparent—a black fin appeared in the water, bearing down on Vansant from the east. Frantically, his father waved for his son to swim to shore, but Vansant spotted the danger too late and when he was fifty yards from the beach he felt a sudden tug and an agonizing pain. As the sea around him turned the color of wine, Vansant reached down to discover that his left leg was gone, severed neatly at the thigh bone.

By now Ott was at his side and dragging him through the water to the safety of the Engelside Hotel where his father desperately tried to stem the bleeding. But it was no use—the wound was too deep—and to his father and young wife's horror Vansant died then and there, the first known victim of a shark attack in the North Atlantic. From that moment on, neither would be able to look at Jersey's Atlantic seaboard without imagining the jaws lurking beneath the surface.

They were not alone. Within fourteen days, four more bathers would also be attacked on the Jersey shore and three would be killed, sparking an obsessive fear of "man-eating" sharks that persists to this day.* It makes little difference that sightings of great whites and other large sharks in the North Atlantic are rare and attacks on swimmers rarer still. Beachgoers now *know* better than to swim too far from shore, and should they become blasé about the risks and dismissive of the menace, there is always a rerun of *Jaws* or an episode of Discovery Channel's *Shark Week* to set them straight. The result is that many children and a fair number of adults are now terrified of playing in the surf, and even those brave enough to venture beyond the breakers *know* to keep a wary eye on the horizon for the telltale sight of a dorsal fin.

AT FIRST GLANCE, the New Jersey shark attacks would seem to have little to do with the Ebola epidemic that engulfed West Africa in 2014 or the Zika epidemic that broke out in Brazil the following year, but they do, for just as in the summer of 1916 most naturalists could not conceive of a shark attack in the cool waters of the North Atlantic, so in the summer of 2014 most infectious disease experts could not imagine that Ebola, a virus previously confined to remote forested regions of Central Africa, might spark an epidemic in a major city in Sierra Leone or Liberia, much less cross the Atlantic to threaten citizens of Europe or the United States. But that is precisely what happened when, shortly before January 2014, Ebola emerged from an unknown animal reservoir and infected a two-year-old boy in the village of Meliandou, in southeastern Guinea, from whence the virus traveled by

---

* The species of shark or sharks responsible for the attacks has never been identified. Some experts believe they were the work of a juvenile great white, *Carcharodon carcharias*; others that they are consistent with the feeding pattern of bull sharks, which are known to favor shallow coastal waters.

road to Conakry, Freetown, and Monrovia, and onward by air to Brussels, London, Madrid, New York, and Dallas.

And something very similar happened in 1997 when a hitherto obscure strain of avian influenza, known as H5N1, which had previously circulated in ducks and other wild waterfowl, suddenly began killing large numbers of poultry in Hong Kong, triggering a worldwide panic about bird flu. The great bird flu scare, of course, was followed by the panic about Severe Acute Respiratory Syndrome (SARS) in 2003, which was followed, in turn, by the 2009 swine flu—an outbreak that began in Mexico and set off an alarm about the threat of a global influenza pandemic that saw the drawdown of stockpiles of antiviral drugs and the production of billions of dollars' worth of vaccines.

Swine flu did not turn into a man-eater—the pandemic killed fewer people globally than common or garden strains of flu have in the United States and the United Kingdom most years—but in the spring of 2009 no one knew that would be the case. Indeed, with disease experts focused on the reemergence of bird flu in Southeast Asia, no one had anticipated the emergence of a novel swine flu virus in Mexico, let alone one with a genetic profile similar to that of the virus of the 1918 "Spanish flu"—a pandemic that is estimated to have killed at least 50 million people worldwide and is considered a byword for viral Armageddon.*

IN THE NINETEENTH CENTURY, medical experts thought that better knowledge of the social and environmental conditions that bred infectious disease would enable them to predict epidemics and, as the Victo-

---

* An epidemic is the rapid spread of infectious disease to a large number of people in a given population within a short period of time. By contrast, a pandemic is an epidemic that has spread across a large region, for instance, multiple countries and continents. This spread may be rapid or may take many months or years. The World Health Organization defines a pandemic simply as the "worldwide spread of a new disease."

rian epidemiologist and sanitarian William Farr put it in 1847, "banish panic." But as advances in bacteriology led to the development of vaccines against typhoid, cholera, and plague, and fear of the great epidemic scourges of the past gradually receded, so other diseases became more visible and new fears took their place. A good example is polio. The month before sharks began attacking bathers on the Jersey shore, a polio epidemic had broken out near the waterfront in South Brooklyn. Investigators from New York's Board of Health immediately blamed the outbreak on recent Italian immigrants from Naples living in crowded, unsanitary tenements in a district known as "Pigtown." As cases of polio multiplied and the papers filled with heartbreaking accounts of dead or paralyzed infants, the publicity prompted hysteria and the flight of wealthy residents (many New Yorkers headed for the Jersey shore). Within weeks, the panic had spread to neighboring states along the eastern seaboard, leading to quarantines, travel bans, and enforced hospitalizations. These hysterical responses partly reflected the then-prevalent medical conviction that polio was a respiratory disease spread by coughs and sneezes and by flies breeding in garbage.*

In his history of poliomyelitis, the epidemiologist John R. Paul describes the epidemic of 1916 as "the high-water mark in attempts at enforcement of isolation and quarantine measures." By the time the epidemic petered out with the cooler weather in December 1916, 27,000 cases and 6,000 deaths had been recorded in twenty-six states, making it the world's then-largest polio outbreak. In New York alone there had been 8,900 cases and 2,400 deaths, a mortality rate of around one child in four.

· The scale of the outbreak made polio appear a peculiarly American problem. But what most Americans did not realize is that a similarly devastating outbreak had visited Sweden five years earlier. During that

---

* In fact, polio is spread principally via the oral-fecal route and nonparalytic polio had been endemic to the United States for several decades prior to 1916.

outbreak, Swedish scientists had repeatedly recovered polio virus from the small intestine of victims—an important step in explicating the true etiology and pathology of the disease. The Swedes also succeeded in culturing the virus in monkeys who had been exposed to secretions from asymptomatic human cases, fueling suspicion about the role of "healthy carriers" in the preservation of the virus between epidemics. However, these insights were ignored by leading American polio experts. The result is that it was not until 1938 that researchers at Yale University would take up the Swedish studies and confirm that asymptomatic carriers frequently excreted the polio virus in their stools and that the virus could survive for up to ten weeks in untreated sewage.

Today, it is recognized that in an era before polio vaccines, the best hope of avoiding the crippling effects of the virus was to contract an immunizing infection in early childhood when polio is less likely to cause severe complications. In this respect, dirt was a mother's friend and exposing babies to water and food contaminated with polio could be considered a rational strategy. By the turn of the nineteenth century, most children from poor immigrant neighborhoods had become immunized in exactly this way. It was children from pristine, middle-class homes and tony areas that were at the greatest risk of developing the paralytic form of the disease—people like Franklin Delano Roosevelt, the thirty-second president of the United States, who escaped polio as a teen, only to contract the disease in 1921 at the age of thirty-nine while holidaying at Campobello island, New Brunswick.

THIS IS A BOOK ABOUT the way that advances in the scientific knowledge of viruses and other infectious pathogens can blind medical researchers to these ecological and immunological insights and the epidemic lurking just around the corner. Ever since the German bacteriologist Robert Koch and his French counterpart, Louis Pasteur, inaugurated the "germ theory" of disease in the 1880s by showing that tuberculosis was a bacterial infection and manufacturing vaccines against anthrax, cholera, and rabies, scientists—and the public health officials who depend on their technologies—have dreamed of defeating the microbes of infectious disease. However, while medical microbiology and the allied sciences of epidemiology, parasitology, zoology, and, more recently, molecular biology, provide new ways of understanding the transmission and spread of novel pathogens and making them visible to clinicians, all too often these sciences and technologies have been found wanting. This is not simply because, as is sometimes argued, microbes are constantly mutating and evolving, outstripping our ability to keep pace with their shifting genetics and transmission patterns. It is also because of the tendency of medical researchers to become prisoners of particular paradigms and theories of disease causation, blinding them to the threats posed by pathogens both known and unknown.

Take influenza, the subject of the first chapter. When the so-called "Spanish flu" emerged in the summer of 1918, during the closing stages of World War I, most physicians assumed it would behave in a similar way to previous flu epidemics and dismissed it as a nuisance. Few thought the pathogen might pose a mortal threat to young adults, much less to soldiers en route to the Allied lines in northern France. This was partly because they had been informed by no less an authority than Koch's protégé, Richard Pfeiffer, that flu was transmitted by a tiny Gram-negative bacterium, and that it would only be a matter of time before American scientists trained in German laboratory methods had manufactured a vaccine against the influenza bacillus, just as they had against cholera, diphtheria, and typhoid. But Pfeiffer and those who put their faith in his experimental methods were wrong: influenza is not a bacterium but a virus that is too small to be seen through the lens of an ordinary optical microscope. Moreover, the virus passed straight through the porcelain filters then used to isolate bacteria commonly found in the nose and throat of influenza sufferers. Although some researchers had begun to suspect that flu might be a "filter-passer," it would be many years before Pfeiffer's misconception would be corrected and influenza's viral etiology divined. In the meantime, many research hours were wasted and millions of young people perished.

However, it would be a mistake to think that simply knowing the identity of a pathogen and the etiology of a disease is sufficient to bring an epidemic under control, for though the presence of an infectious microbe may be a necessary condition for ill health, it is rarely sufficient. Microbes interact with our immune systems in various ways, and a pathogen that causes disease in one person, may leave another unaffected or only mildly inconvenienced. Indeed, many bacterial and viral infections can lie dormant in tissue and cells for decades before being reactivated by some extrinsic event or process, whether it be coinfection with another microbe, a sudden shock to the system due to an external stress, or the waning of immunity with old age. More importantly, by taking specific microbial predators as our focus we risk missing the bigger picture. For instance, the Ebola virus may be one of the deadliest pathogens known to humankind, but it is only when tropical rain forests are degraded by clear-cutting, dislodging from their roosts the bats in which the virus is presumed to reside between epidemics, or when people hunt chimpanzees infected with the virus and butcher them for the table, that Ebola risks spilling over into humans. And it is only when the blood-borne infection is amplified by poor hospital hygiene practices that it is likely to spread to the wider community and have a chance of reaching urban areas. In such circumstances, it is worth keeping in mind the view expressed by George Bernard Shaw in *The Doctor's Dilemma*, namely that "The characteristic microbe of a disease might be a symptom instead of a cause." Indeed, updating Shaw's axiom for the present day, we might say that infectious diseases nearly always have wider environmental and social causes. Unless and until we take account of the ecological, immunological, and behavioral factors that govern the emergence and spread of novel pathogens, our knowledge of such microbes and their connection to disease is bound to be partial and incomplete.

In fairness, there have always been medical researchers prepared to take a more nuanced view of our complex interactions with microbes. For instance, writing at the height of the antibiotics revolution fifty years ago, the Rockefeller researcher René Dubos railed against short-term technological fixes for medical problems. At a time when most of his colleagues took the conquest of infectious disease for granted and assumed that the eradication of the common bacterial causes of infection was just around the corner, Dubos, who had isolated the first commercial antibiotic in 1939 and knew what he was talking about, sounded a note of caution against the prevailing medical hubris. Comparing man to the "sorcerer's apprentice," he argued that medical science had set in motion "potentially destructive forces" that might one day usurp the dreams of a medical utopia. "Modern man believes that he has achieved almost completely mastery over the natural forces which molded his evolution in the past and that he can now control his own biological and cultural destiny," wrote Dubos. "But this may be an illusion. Like all other living things, he is part of an immensely complex ecological system and is bound to all its components by innumerable links." Instead, Dubos argued that complete freedom from disease was a "mirage" and that "at some unpredictable time and in some unforeseeable manner nature will strike back."

Yet for all that Dubos's writings were hugely popular with the American public in the 1960s, his warnings of a coming disease Armageddon were largely ignored by his scientific colleagues. The result was that when, shortly after Dubos's death in February 1982, the Centers for Disease Control and Prevention (CDC) coined the acronym, AIDS, to describe an unusual autoimmune condition that had suddenly appeared in the homosexual community in Los Angeles and was now spreading to other segments of the population, it took the medical world by surprise. But really the CDC shouldn't have been surprised because something very similar had happened just eight years earlier when an outbreak of atypical pneumonia among a group of war veterans who had attended an American Legion convention at a luxury hotel in Philadelphia sparked widespread hysteria as epidemiologists scrambled to identify the "Philly Killer" (the outbreak initially flummoxed the CDC's disease detectives and it took a microbiologist to identify the pathogen, *Legionella pneumophila*, a tiny bacterium that thrives in aquatic environments, including the cooling towers of hotels). That year, 1976, saw not only a panic over Legionnaires' disease, but a panic over the sudden emergence of a new strain of swine flu at a US Army base in New Jersey—an emergence event for which the CDC and public health officials were likewise unprepared and that would eventually result in the needless vaccination of millions of Americans. And something very similar happened again in 2003 when an elderly Chinese professor of nephrology checked into the Metropole Hotel in Hong Kong, igniting cross-border outbreaks of a severe respiratory illness that was initially blamed on the H5N1 avian influenza virus but which we now know to have been due to a novel coronavirus* associated with SARS. In that case, a pandemic was averted by some nifty microbiological detective work and unprecedented cooperation between networks of scientists sharing information, but it was a close call, and since then we have seen several more unanticipated—and initially misdiagnosed—emergence events.

This is a book about these events and processes, and the reasons why, despite our best efforts to predict and prepare for them, they continue to take us by surprise. Some of these epidemic histories, such as the panic over the 2014–2016 Ebola epidemic or the hysteria over AIDS in the 1980s, will be familiar to readers; others, such as

---

* Coronoaviruses primarily infect the respiratory and gastrointestinal tracts of mammals and are thought to be the cause of up to one-third of common colds.

the pneumonic plague outbreak that erupted in the Mexican quarter of Los Angeles in 1924, or the great "parrot fever" panic that swept the United States a few months after the Wall Street Crash, less so. Whether familiar or not, however, each of these epidemics illustrates how quickly the received medical wisdom can be overturned by the emergence of new pathogens and how, in the absence of laboratory knowledge and effective vaccines and treatment drugs, such epidemics have an unusual power to provoke panic, hysteria, and dread.

Far from banishing panic, better medical knowledge and surveillance of infectious disease can also sow new fears, making people hyperaware of epidemic threats of which they had previously been ignorant. The result is that just as lifeguards now scan the sea for dorsal fins in the hope of forewarning bathers, so the World Health Organization (WHO) routinely scans the internet for reports of unusual disease outbreaks and tests for mutations that might signal the emergence of the next pandemic virus. To some extent this hypervigilance makes sense. But the price we pay is a permanent state of anxiety about the next Big One. It's not a question *if* Apocalypse will occur, we're repeatedly told, but *when*. In this febrile atmosphere it is not surprising that public health experts sometimes get it wrong and press the panic button when, in reality, no panic is warranted. Or, as in the case of the West African Ebola epidemic, misread the threat entirely.

To be sure, the media plays its part in these processes—after all, nothing sells like fear—but while 24/7 cable news channels and social media help to fuel the panic, hysteria, and stigma associated with infectious disease outbreaks, journalists and bloggers are, for the most part, merely messengers. I argue that by alerting us to new sources of infection and framing particular behaviors as "risky," it is medical science—and the science of epidemiology in particular—that is the ultimate source of these irrational and often prejudicial judgments. No one would wish to deny that better knowledge of the epidemiology and causes of infectious diseases has led to huge advances in preparedness for epidemics, or that technological advances in medicine have brought about immense improvements in health and well-being; nevertheless, we should recognize that this knowledge is constantly giving birth to new fears and anxieties.

Each epidemic canvassed in this book illustrates a different aspect of this process, showing how in each case the outbreak undermined confidence in the dominant medical and scientific paradigm, highlighting the dangers of overreliance on particular technologies at the expense of wider ecological insights into disease causation. Drawing on sociological and philosophical insights into the construction of scientific knowledge, I argue that what was "known" before the emergence event—that water towers and air conditioning systems ("Legionnaires' disease") *don't* present a risk to hotel guests and the occupants of hospitals, that Ebola *doesn't* circulate in West Africa and *can't* reach a major city, that Zika is a relatively harmless mosquito-borne illness—was shown to be false; and I explain how, in each case, the epidemics would spark much retrospective soul-searching about "known knowns" and "unknown unknowns" and what scientists and public health experts should do to avoid such epistemological blind spots in the future.[*]

The epidemics canvassed in this book also underline the key role played by environmental, social, and cultural factors in changing patterns of disease prevalence and emergence. Recalling Dubos's insights into the ecology of pathogens, I argue that most cases of disease emergence can be traced to the disturbance of ecological equilibriums or alterations to the environments in which pathogens habitually reside. This is especially true of animal origin or zoonotic viruses such as Ebola, but it is also true of commensal bacteria such as streptococci,

---

[*] The concepts of "known knowns" and "unknown unknowns" were infamously introduced into public discourse by the former US secretary of defense Donald Rumsfeld at a Pentagon news conference in 2002 (see endnotes for further discussion).

the main cause of community-acquired pneumonias. The natural host of Ebola is thought to be a fruit bat. However, though antibodies to Ebola have been found in various species of bats indigenous to Africa, live virus has never been recovered from any of them. The reason, most likely, is that as with other viruses that are adapted to their hosts as a result of long evolutionary association, the Ebola virus is quickly cleared from the bloodstream by the bat's immune system, but not before, presumably, it has been transmitted to another bat. The result is that the virus circulates continually in bat populations, without leading to the destruction of either. A similar process occurs with pathogens that have evolved so as to infect only humans, such as measles and polio, with a first infection in childhood usually resulting in a mild illness, after which the subject recovers and enjoys lifelong immunity. However, every now and again these states of immunological balance are disrupted. This may occur naturally if, for instance, sufficient numbers of children escape infection in childhood to cause herd immunity to wane, or if the virus suddenly mutates, as occurs frequently with influenza, leading to the circulation of a new strain against which people have little or no immunity. But it can also occur when we accidentally interpose ourselves between the virus and its natural host. This is presumably what happened with Ebola in 2014 when children in Meliandou began taunting long-tailed bats roosting in a tree stump in the middle of their village. And it is thought that something very similar may have prompted the spillover of the HIV progenitor virus from chimpanzees to humans in the Congo in the 1950s. Tracing the precise genesis of these epidemics is the subject of ongoing research. In the case of AIDS, there is little doubt that the inauguration of steamship travel on the Congo River at the turn of the twentieth century and the construction of new roads and railways in the colonial period were important contributing factors, as was the greed of loggers and timber companies. However, social and cultural factors also played a part: were it not for the practice of consuming bushmeat and widespread prostitution near the camps supplying labor to the rail and timber companies, the virus would probably not have spread so widely or been amplified so rapidly. Similarly, were it not for entrenched cultural beliefs and customs in West Africa—in particular, people's adherence to traditional burial rituals and their distrust of scientific medicine—it is unlikely that Ebola would have morphed into a major regional epidemic, let alone a global health crisis.

However, perhaps the most important insight medical history can bring is of the long association between epidemics and war. Ever since Pericles ordered Athenians to sit out the Spartan siege of their harbor city in 430 BC, wars have been seen as progenitors of deadly outbreaks of infectious disease (this was certainly the case in West Africa in 2014, where decades of civil war and armed conflict had left Liberia and Sierra Leone with weak and underresourced health systems). Though the pathogen responsible for the plague of Athens has never been identified and perhaps never will be (candidates include anthrax, smallpox, typhus, and malaria), there is little doubt that the decisive factor was the crowding of upwards of 300,000 Athenians and refugees from Attica behind the Long Walls of the Greek city. That confinement created the ideal conditions for the amplification of the virus—if virus it was—turning Athens into a charnel house (as Thucydides informs us, as there were no houses to receive the refugees from the countryside "they had to be lodged at the hot season of the year in stifling cabins, where the mortality raged without restraint"). The result was that by the third wave of the disease in 426 BC, Athens's population had been reduced by between one-quarter and one-third.

In the case of the Athenian plague, for reasons that are unclear, the disease does not appear to have affected the Spartans, or spread far beyond the borders of Attica. But 2,000 years ago, towns and cities were more isolated and there was far less passage of people and pathogens between countries and continents. Unfortunately, this is not the case today. Thanks to global trade and travel, novel viruses and their vectors are continually crossing borders and international time zones, and in each place they encounter a different mix of ecological and immunological conditions. This was nowhere more true than during World War I, when the congregation of tens of thousands of young American recruits in training camps on the eastern seaboard of the United States and their subsequent passage to and from Europe provided the ideal conditions for the deadliest outbreak of pandemic disease in history.

CHAPTER I

THE BLUE DEATH

"Ordinariness is what strikes one first about the town of Oran."
—ALBERT CAMUS, *The Plague*

I
t was an unassuming village, much like any you would have encountered on a rural tour of New England in 1917. Blink and you might have missed it. Set in drab scrubland thirty-five miles northwest of Boston, Ayer comprised fewer than three hundred cottage-like dwellings, plus a church and a couple of stores. Indeed, were it not for the fact that the village sat at the junction of the Boston and Maine and Worcester and Nashua railroads and boasted two stations, there would have been little to recommend it. But in the spring of 1917, as America prepared to go to war and military planners began looking for suitable sites to train thousands of men responding to the draft, those railroad stations and empty fields marked Ayer out as special, unusual even. Perhaps that is why in May 1917 someone in Washington, DC stuck a pin with a red flag in a map of Lowell County, Massachusetts, and designated Ayer as the site of the cantonment of the new Seventy-Sixth Division of the US Army.

In early June leases were signed with owners of some 9,000 acres of treeless "sprout" land adjacent to the Nashua River, and two weeks later engineers arrived to transform the site into a camp fit for Major General John Pershing's doughboys. In the space of just ten weeks, engineers constructed 1,400 buildings, installed 2,200 shower baths, and laid sixty miles of heating pipes. Measuring seven miles by two, the cantonment contained its own restaurant, bakery, theater, fourteen huts for reading and fraternizing, plus a post and telegraph office. Arriving from Ayer—a short half-mile walk that led across the tracks of the Fitchburg railroad—the first sight to greet newly drafted men was the huge YMCA auditorium and the barracks of the 301st engineers. To the right lay the barracks of the 301st, 302nd, and 303rd infantry divisions, and nearby, those for the field artillery, depot brigade, and machine-gun brigade. Beyond that lay fields for practicing drill and bayoneting skills, and an eight-hundred-bed hospital, also run by the YMCA. In all, the cantonment was capable of housing 30,000 men. But over the next few weeks, as raw recruits arrived from Maine, Rhode Island, Connecticut, New York, Minnesota, and as far south as Florida, the rough wooden barracks would be filled with in excess of 40,000 men, forcing engineers to erect tents for the overflow. In recognition of its importance to the northeastern military command, the cantonment was named Camp Devens in honor of General Charles Devens, a Boston lawyer turned Civil War commander whose Union troops were the first to occupy Richmond after its fall in 1865. As Roger Batchelder, a propagandist for the War Department, put it, admiring Camp Devens from a hill outside Ayer in December 1917, the cantonment resembled nothing so much as a "huge city of soldiers." What the observer did not say was that Devens also represented an unprecedented immunological experiment. Never before had so many men from so many different walks of life—factory workers and farmhands, machinists and college graduates—been brought together in such numbers and forced to live cheek by jowl.

Camp Devens was not the only camp to be hastily constructed that summer, nor was it the biggest. In all, draftees destined for the American Expeditionary Force would be sent for training to forty large camps across the United States. Some, such as Camp Funston, built on the site of a former cavalry station at Fort Riley, Kansas, accommodated as many as 55,000 men. Meanwhile, on the opposite side of the

Atlantic at Etaples in northern France, the British had constructed an even larger facility. Built on low-lying meadows adjoining the railway line from Boulogne to Paris, Etaples had bunks for up to 100,000 British and Imperial troops and hospital beds for 22,000. In the course of the war, it is estimated that one million soldiers passed through Etaples en route to the Somme and other battlegrounds.

Nor were the facilities at many of these camps always as good as war supporters suggested. Indeed, in many cases mobilization had been so swift that engineers had been unable to complete the construction of hospitals and other medical facilities in time, and barracks were often so drafty that men were forced to huddle around stoves in the evening to keep warm and to sleep in extra layers of clothing at night. Some, such as Batchelder, saw this as a way of toughening recruits and preparing them for the hardships of trench warfare in northern France. "At Ayer it is cold, but . . . the cold weather is exhilarating; it inures the men who have always lived in hot houses to the out-door life." However, others criticized the War Department for selecting a site so far north, saying it would have been better if Devens had been located in the South where the weather was more hospitable.

In truth, the principal danger was not the cold so much as the overcrowding. By bringing together men from so many different immunological backgrounds and forcing them to live at close quarters for weeks on end, the mobilization greatly increased the risk of communicable diseases being spread from one to another. Wars have always been incubators of disease, of course. What was different in 1917 was the scale of the call-up and the intermixing of men raised in very different ecological settings. In urban areas, where populations are denser, the chances of being exposed to measles or common respiratory pathogens, such as *Streptococcus pneumoniae* and *Staphylococcus aureus*, is far higher and usually occurs in childhood. By contrast, in an era before cars and buses, when children raised in rural areas tended to be educated at grade schools close to their homes, many avoided exposure to measles. Nor would many have been exposed to *Streptococcus pyrogenes* and other hemolyticus bacteria that cause "strep throat." The result was that as the US Army grew from 378,000 in April 1917 to a force of 1.5 million by the turn of 1918 (by the war's end, in November 1918, the combined strength of the US Army and Navy would be 4.7 million), epidemics of measles and pneumonia erupted at camps all along the eastern seaboard, as well as in several southern states.

Prior to the introduction of antibiotics, pneumonia accounted for roughly one-quarter of all deaths in the United States. These pneumonias could be triggered by bacteria, viruses, fungi, or parasites, but by far the largest source of community-acquired outbreaks were pneumococcal bacteria (*Steptococcus pneumoniae*). Under the microscope these pneumococcal bacteria resemble any other streptococcus. However, one of S. pneumoniae's unusual features is that it possesses a polysaccharide (sugar) capsule that protects it from drying out in air or being ingested by phagocytes, one of the immune system's principal cellular defenses. Indeed, in moist sputum in a darkened room, pneumococci can survive on surfaces for up to ten days.

Worldwide, there are more than eighty subtypes of pneumococcal bacteria, each one differing from the others in terms of the constitution of its capsule. For the most part, these bacteria reside in the nose and throat without causing illness, but if a person's immune system is impaired or compromised by another disease, such as measles or influenza, the bacteria can get the upper hand, triggering potentially fatal lung infections. Typically, such infections begin as an inflammation of the alveoli, the microscopic sacs that absorb oxygen in the lungs. As the bacteria invade the alveoli, they are pursued by leukocytes and other immune cells, as well as fluids containing proteins and enzymes. As the air sacs fill they become "consolidated" with material, making it harder for them to transfer oxygen to the blood. Usually, this consolidation appears in patches surrounding the bronchi, the passages which branch from the bronchus, the tube that carries air from the trachea into the right and left lungs. When this consolidation is localized it is known as bronchopneumonia. However, in more severe infections, this consolidation can spread across entire lobes (the right lung has three, the left two) turning the lungs into a solid, liverlike mass. The effect on lung tissue is dramatic. A healthy lung is spongy and porous and a good conductor of sound. When a doctor listens to the breathing of a healthy patient through a stethoscope he or she should hear very little. By contrast, a congested lung conducts breathing sounds to the wall of the chest, resulting in rattling or cracking sounds known as rales.

In the late Victorian and Edwardian period, pneumonia was perhaps the most feared disease after tuberculosis and nearly always fatal, particularly in the elderly or those whose immune systems were compromised by other diseases. Prominent victims included the ninth president of the United States, William Henry Harrison, who died one month after his inauguration in 1841, and the Confederate general Thomas Jonathan "Stonewall" Jackson, who died of complications of pneumonia eight days after being wounded at the Battle of Chancellorsville in 1863. Little wonder then that Sir William Osler, the so-called father of modern American medicine, dubbed pneumonia the "Captain of the Men of Death."

When contracted in childhood measles usually results in a rash and high fever accompanied by a violent cough and sensitivity to light, but in the case of the camp-acquired measles cases the symptoms were far more severe. The outbreaks produced the highest infection rates the army had seen in ninety-seven years and were often accompanied by an aggressive bronchopneumonia. The result was that between September 1917 and March 1918, more than 30,000 American troops were hospitalized with pneumonia, nearly all as a result of complications of measles, and some 5,700 died. The extent of the outbreaks astonished even battled-hardened doctors, such as Victor Vaughan, the dean of the University of Michigan's School of Medicine and a veteran of the Spanish-American War. "Not a troop train came into Camp Wheeler (near Macon, Georgia) in the fall of 1917 without bringing one to six cases of measles already in the eruptive stage," he wrote. "These men had brought the infection from their homes and had distributed its seed at the state encampment and on the train. No power on earth could stop the spread of measles through a camp under these conditions. Cases developed, from one hundred to five hundred a day, and the infection continued as long as there was susceptible material in the camp."

By the spring of 1918 the War Department was being lambasted by Congress for shipping recruits to training camps before facilities were fully ready and under conditions that failed to meet basic standards of public health, and by July the department had appointed a pneumonia commission to investigate the unusual prevalence of the disease in the large cantonments. The commission read like a future who's who of American medicine, and included Eugenie L. Opie, the future dean of Washington University School of Medicine; Francis G. Blake, who would go on to become professor of internal medicine at Yale University; and Thomas Rivers, who would become one of the world's leading virologists and director of the Rockefeller University hospital in New York. Assisting them in the surgeon general's office with the rank of commanders were Victor Vaughan and William H. Welch, the dean of Johns Hopkins School of Medicine and then the most famous pathologist and bacteriologist in America, and Rufus Cole, the first director of the Rockefeller University Hospital and a specialist in pneumococcal disease. Together with his assistant Oswald Avery, Cole would direct laboratory investigations of the pneumonia outbreaks and train medical officers in the correct techniques for culturing the bacteria and making serums and vaccines. Meanwhile, keeping a watch over their endeavors would be Simon Flexner, the head of Rockefeller Institute and a former student and protégé of Welch.

WHILE AMERICAN PHYSICIANS were worrying about camp-acquired measles and pneumonia cases, medics in the British Army were becoming
concerned about another respiratory disease. Labeled "purulent bronchitis" for want of a better term, the disease had broken out at Etaples in
the bitterly cold winter of 1917, and by February 156 soldiers were dead.
The initial stages resembled ordinary lobar pneumonia—a high fever
and the expectoration of blood-streaked sputum. But these symptoms
soon gave way to a racing pulse accompanied by the discharge of thick
pale yellow dollops of pus, suggesting bronchitis. In half these cases
death from "lung block" followed soon after.

Another striking feature was cyanosis. This condition occurs when
a patient becomes breathless because the lungs can no longer transfer
oxygen efficiently to the blood and is characterized by a dusky purple-
blue discoloration of the face, lips, and ears (it is oxygen that turns
blood in the arteries red). However, in the case of the Etaples patients,
their breathlessness was so acute that they tore off their bedclothes in
distress. At autopsy, the pathologist, William Rolland, was shocked to
find a thick, yellowish pus blocking the bronchi. In the larger bronchi, the pus was mixed with air, but when he cut a section through
the smaller tubes he wrote, "the pus exudes spontaneously . . . with
little or no admixture of air." This explained why the attempt to relieve
patients' symptoms by giving them piped oxygen had been of little
use. Etaples was not the only army camp where this peculiar disease
appeared. In March 1917 a similar outbreak had occurred at Aldershot, "The Home of the British Army," in southern England. Once
again the disease proved fatal to half those it infected, the signature
feature being the exudation of a yellowish pus followed by breathlessness and cyanosis. In the cyanosed patients, physicians noted, "no
treatment that we have been able to devise appears to do any good."
To some, the short shallow breathing recalled the "effects of gas poi-

soning," but later the bacteriologists and pathologists who examined the Aldershot and Etaples cases became convinced it had been a type of influenza. Flu had long been recognized as trigger for bronchial infections. During influenza epidemics and the seasonal outbreaks of the disease which occurred every fall and winter, epidemiologists were accustomed to seeing a spike in respiratory deaths, particularly among the very young or elderly sections of the population. But for young adults and those below the age of seventy, flu was considered more of a nuisance than a mortal threat to life, and convalescents were frequently viewed with suspicion.

WE MAY NEVER KNOW whether the outbreaks at Etaples and Aldershot were flu, but in March 1918 another unusual respiratory outbreak visited a large army camp—this time at Camp Funston in Kansas. Initially, physicians thought they were seeing another wave of camp-acquired pneumonias, but they soon revised their opinion.

The first casualty was supposedly the camp cook. On March 4, he woke with a splitting headache and aches in his neck and back and reported to the base hospital. Soon, one hundred other members of the 164th Depot Brigade had joined him, and by the third week in March more than 1,200 men were on the sick list, forcing Fort Riley's chief medical officer to requisition a hangar adjacent to the hospital for the overflow. The illness resembled classic influenza: chills followed by high fever, sore throat, headache, and abdominal pains. However, many patients were so incapacitated that they found it impossible to stand up; hence the malady's nickname, "knock-me-down fever." Most of the men recovered within three to five days, but, disturbingly, several went on to develop severe pneumonias. Unlike the pneumonias after measles, which tended to localize in the bronchi, these postinfluenzal pneumonias frequently extended to the entire lobe of a lung. In all, such lobar pneumonias had developed in 237 men, roughly one-fifth of those hospitalized, and by May there had been 75 deaths. As Opie and Rivers discovered the following July when the pneumonia commission eventually arrived to conduct an investigation, there were other disturbing features, too: after the initial epidemic had petered out in March there had been further outbreaks in April and May, each one corresponding to the arrival of a new group of draftees. Not only that, but men transferred to camps in the East appeared to carry the disease with them, and when many of these same men joined the American Expeditionary Force and mingled freely with soldiers sailing for Europe, they sparked further outbreaks on board Atlantic troopships. The pattern continued when the transports arrived at Brest, the main disembarkation point for American troops, and disgorged their cargo. "Epidemic of acute infectious fever, nature unknown," reported a medical officer at a US Army hospital in Bordeaux on April 15. As at Funston, the initial cases were mild but by June thousands of Allied troops were being hospitalized, and by August alarm was mounting. "These successive outbreaks tended to be progressively more severe both in character and extent, which would speak for an increasing virulence of the causative agent," observed Alan M. Chesney, a medical officer at an AEF artillery training camp in Valdahon.

Chesney's was a rare example of concern. In the summer of 1918 no one had experienced a pandemic of influenza for twenty-eight years. Compared to typhus, a deadly blood-borne disease spread by lice that lived in soldiers' clothing, or the septicemia that bred in gunshot and shrapnel wounds, influenza was a trifling infection from the point of view of army medical officers. Civilian physicians regarded flu with similar disdain, particularly the British, who had long considered influenza a suspect Italian word for a bad cold or catarrh.* Besides, after nearly five years of brutal trench warfare which had already

---

* *Influenza* derives from the Latinate Italian phrase *influenza coeli*, meaning "influence of the heavens."

claimed the lives of tens of thousands of Europeans, and with two million Allied troops now dug in in northern France and Flanders, officers had more pressing issues on their minds. "Quite 1/3 of the Batt. and about 30 officers are smitten with the Spanish Flu," the poet Wilfred Owen informed his mother, Susan, disdainfully in a letter from a British Army camp in Scarborough, North Yorkshire, in June. "The thing is much too common for me to take part in. I have quite decided not to! Imagine the work that falls on unaffected officers."

Owen was wrong to be so complacent. Between the summer of 1918 and the spring of 1919, tens of thousands of soldiers and millions of civilians would be mown down by Spanish flu (so-called because Spain was the only country not to censor reports of the spreading epidemic) as the disease ricocheted between America and northern Europe before engulfing the entire globe. In the United States alone, some 675,000 Americans would perish in the successive waves of flu; in France, perhaps as many as 400,000; in Britain, 228,000. World-wide, the death toll from the Spanish flu pandemic has been estimated at 50 million—five times as many as died in the fighting in World War One and 10 million more than AIDS has killed in thirty years.

One reason Owen and others were so relaxed about influenza was that in 1918, medical scientists were confident that they knew how the disease was transmitted. After all, in 1892 Richard Pfeiffer, the son-in-law of Robert Koch, the German "father" of bacteriology, had announced that he had identified the disease's "exciting cause," a tiny Gram-negative bacterium he dubbed *Bacillus influenzae*. Pfeiffer's "discovery" came at the height of the so-called Russian influenza pandemic and made headline news around the world, fueling expectations that it would only be a matter of time before scientists trained in German laboratory techniques had produced a vaccine. Never mind that other researchers were not always able to isolate "Pfeiffer's bacillus," as the bacterium was popularly known, from the throat washings and bronchial expectorations of influenza patients. Or that it was notoriously difficult to cultivate the bacteria on artificial media and it often took several attempts to grow colonies of sufficient size so that the small, spherical, and colorless bodies could be visualized through a microscope using special dyes. Or that despite inoculating monkeys with the bacillus, Pfeiffer and his Berlin colleague, Shibashuro Kitasato, had so far been unable to transfer the disease, thereby failing the test of Koch's fourth postulate. As far as most medical authorities were concerned, Pfeiffer's bacillus *was* the etiological agent of influenza and that was that. Rare was the man of science who dared to challenge the authority of Koch and his disciples by expressing unease at the failure to find the bacillus in each and every case of influenza.

Perhaps that explains why, on arriving at Camp Funston in July, Opie, Blake, and Rivers had ignored the fact that researchers had failed to find *Bacillus influenzae* in 77 percent of the pneumonia cases, or that the bacillus had also been isolated from the mouths of one-third of the healthy men, i.e., those who had *not* shown any signs or symptoms of influenza.[*] Instead, they tried to make sense of the higher pneumonia attack rates observed among African American draftees from Louisiana and Mississippi, an incidence they attributed to racial differences between white and "colored" troops. This was despite observing that the units that had suffered most severely from postinfluenzal pneumonias were the ones that were new to the camp and who had only been at Fort Riley for three to six months, and that a greater proportion of the African American draftees came from rural areas. For the most part, the survey was dull, repetitive work and Blake soon found himself longing for a change of scene. As he complained to his wife on August 9, "No letter from my beloved for two days. No cool days, no cool nights, no drinks, no movies, no dances, no club, no pretty women, no shower bath, no poker, no people, no fun, no joy, no nothing save heat and blistering sun and scorching winds and

* Today the bacillus is referred to as *Hemophilus influenzae*.

sweat and dust and thirst and long and stifling nights and working all hours and lonesomeness and general hell—that's Fort Riley, Kansas."

Very soon Opie, Blake, and Rivers would get orders to leave Kansas, only to be thrust into a far worse hell when they found themselves in the midst of a raging epidemic of influenza and pneumonia at Camp Pike, Arkansas. They were spared the worst hell of all, however.

≫≪

IN AUGUST 1918, Clifton Skillings, a twenty-three-year-old farmer from Ripley, Maine, boarded a southbound Boston train. Like thousands of other American men of fighting age, Skillings had received his draft papers a few weeks earlier and had now been ordered to report for duty to Camp Devens. Alighting at Ayer, he fell into step with other draftees dressed in their Sunday best and began striding toward the camp, with a trooper on horseback leading the way. To the eyes of the Boston men, Ayer was a "hick town." Whether Skillings thought it so he does not say, but to judge by his letters and his postcards he did not care particularly for the food. "We had your beans at noon but they are not like the beans you get at home," he complained to his family on August 24. "It makes me think of mixing up dog food." Skillings immediately fell in with a group from Skowhegan, Maine, but was amazed to learn that the camp included men from midwestern states such as Minnesota. "There is a good many thousand men in this campground. It seems awful funny to see nothing but men . . . I wish you folks could come in & look around." Four weeks later the size of the camp and the quality of food is the least of his concerns, however. "Lots of the boys are sick and in the hospital," he wrote home on September 23. "It is a disease. Some [thing] like the Gripp . . . I don't think I will get it."

It's not known where the fall wave of influenza originated. It could have been incubating in America over the summer, but more likely it was introduced by troops returning from Europe. From an ecologi-

cal point of view, northern France was a vast biological experiment—
a place where large masses of men from two continents converged
and mingled freely with men from a host of other nations, including
Indian soldiers from the Punjab, African regiments from Nigeria and
Sierra Leone, Chinese "coolies," and Indochinese laborers from Vietnam, Laos, and Cambodia. One theory is that the second wave began
with an outbreak at a coaling station in Sierra Leone at the end of
August, from whence it spread rapidly to other West African countries
and to Europe via British naval vessels. Another is that the bug was
already in Europe, hence the prepandemic waves recorded in Copenhagen and other northern European cities in July.

In the United States, the fall wave had first announced itself
toward the end of August at Commonwealth Pier in Boston, one of
the main entry points for returning AEF troops, when several sailors
were suddenly taken ill. By August 29, fifty had been transferred
to the Chelsea Naval Hospital, where they came under the care of
Lieutenant Commander Milton Rosenau, a former director of the US
Public Health Service's Hygienic Laboratory and member of Harvard
Medical School. Rosenau isolated the sailors in an effort to contain
the outbreak, but by early September US naval stations in Newport,
Rhode Island, and New London, Connecticut were also reporting
significant numbers of influenza cases. At around the same time,
Devens saw an increase in pneumonia cases. Then, on September 7,
a soldier from Company B, 42nd infantry, was admitted to the base
hospital with "epidemic meningitis." In fact, his symptoms—runny
nose, sore throat, and inflammation of the nasal passages—were consistent with influenza, and when the following day twelve more men
from the same company fell ill with similar symptoms, doctors had
no hesitation in labeling it a "mild" form of Spanish influenza. It
would not remain mild for long.

When a parasitic organism meets a susceptible host for the first
time, it triggers an arms race between the pathogen and the host's

immune system. Having never encountered the pathogen before, the immune system is initially blindsided and takes time to mobilize its defenses and launch a counterattack. With nothing to stop it, the pathogen tears through the host's tissue, invading cells and multiplying at will. At this stage, the parasite resembles a child with a tantrum. With no one and nothing to discipline it, its tantrum can easily escalate and its behavior can become increasingly virulent. Eventually, in the most extreme cases of all, its rage may become all-consuming. This is usually bad news for the host. From a Darwinian point of view, however, the parasite does not want to kill its host; its primary objective is to survive long enough to escape and infect a new susceptible. In other words, the death of the host is a bad strategy for a parasite, an "accident" of biology if you will. A far better survival strategy over the long term is to evolve in the other direction, toward avirulence, resulting in an infection that is mild or barely detectable in the host. But in order for that to happen, the immune system must first find a way of taming the parasite.

It did not take long for the infection to spread from the 42nd infantry to adjacent barracks, and when it did, the flu was nothing like the "mild" spring wave. It was explosive. By September 10 more than five hundred men had been admitted to the base hospital at Devens. Within four days, those numbers had tripled, and on September 15 a further 705 were admitted. The next three days were the worst, however. On September 16 medical orderlies had to find beds for a further 1,189 men and the following day beds for 2,200 more. The pneumonia cases began to mount soon afterward, but they were nothing like the bronchopneumonias associated with measles. They resembled more severe versions of the lobar pneumonias that had developed in some of the flu cases at Camp Funston in the spring. "These men start with what appears to be an ordinary attack of *LaGrippe* or Influenza, and when brought to the Hosp. they very rapidly develop the most vicious type of Pneumonia that has ever been seen," recalled a Scottish physician named Roy who was present when pneumonia ripped through the wards. "Two hours after admission they have the Mahogany spots over the cheek bones, and a few hours later you can begin to see the Cyanosis extending from their ears and spreading all over the face, until it is hard to distinguish the coloured men from the white. . . . One could stand it to see, one, two or twenty men die, but to see these poor devils dropping like flies . . . is horrible."

As the writer John Barry noted in his book *The Great Influenza*, in 1918 these cyanoses were so extreme that victims' entire bodies would take on a dark purple hue, sparking "rumours that the disease was not influenza, but the Black Death." British Army medical officers, many, like Welch and Vaughan, experienced civilian physicians and pathologists who had taken military commissions at the outset of war, were similarly impressed by these cyanotic cases and, struck by the resemblance with the cyanoses seen at Etaples and Aldershot in the winter of 1917, commissioned an artist from the Royal Academy to paint patients in the last throes of illness. The artist labeled the final stage "heliotrope cyanosis" after the deep blue flowers of the same name.

As concerns about measles and pneumonia had grown over the summer, the surgeon general's office in Washington had kept Welch, Vaughan, and Cole busy. They were sent to make an inspection of Camp Wheeler, near Macon, Georgia, and other camps in the South. On leaving Macon in early September, Welch had suggested they stop at the Mountain Meadows Inn, a fashionable retreat in Asheville, North Carolina. A portly man famous for his love of cigars and gourmet dining, Welch was now in his late sixties and, except for a strip of white around the ears, almost completely bald. To offset the absence of hair on top, he sported a fashionable goatee and moustache, which were also white. To some this gave him the appearance of an elder statesman—an impression underscored by his reputation for being an aloof and distracted teacher. But that was the older Welch. In his youth his imagination had been fired by reports from Germany of the advances being made in the understanding of disease processes using the microscope and new laboratory methods, and in 1876 he had set sail for Leipzig to work with Carl Ludwig, then the foremost experimental pathologist in the world. From Ludwig, Welch learned that "the most important lesson for a microscopist [was] not to be satisfied with loose thinking and half proofs . . . but to observe closely and carefully facts." The experience made an indelible impression and, on his return to the United States, Welch set about conveying the principles and techniques he had acquired in Europe to a new generation of American medical students, first at Bellevue Medical College, New York, and later at Johns Hopkins, the university that, more than any other American institution, is credited with creating a new paradigm for medical education in the United States. There, to contemporaries such as William Osler and William Steward Halstead, Welch was considered a bon vivant whose favorite pastimes were swimming, carnival rides, and five-dessert dinners in Atlantic City. But for all that they might tease the confirmed bachelor by referring to him as "Popsy," they also recognized that few could equal Welch's skills as an anatomist. When Welch cared to, he could also awe his students with his intellect and knowledge of art and culture. As Simon Flexner, who went on to write a biography of his former teacher, recalled, Welch's technique was initially to ignore his students and leave them to their own devices in the laboratory. But on rare evenings when he invited promising students to dine with him, "a spell fell over the room as the quiet voice talked on, and the young men, some of them already a little round-shouldered from too much peering into the microscope . . . resolved to go to art galleries, to hear music, to read the masterpieces of literature about which Welch discoursed so excitingly."

Welch and his colleagues used their stay in North Carolina to go over what they had learned during their tour of the South. The consensus was that a better understanding of the immunity of newly drafted men held the key to understanding the measles and pneumonia outbreaks. The Meadows Inn "is a delightful, restful, quiet place," Welch observed on September 19. It would be the last respite the group would enjoy for some time.

Two days later they were back in Washington, DC, but no sooner had they alighted at Union Station than they were informed that Devens had been struck by Spanish influenza and they were to proceed immediately to Ayer. The scene that confronted them there was shocking and difficult to comprehend. By now the base hospital was overflowing with patients and care was almost nonexistent. More than 6,000 men were crammed into the 800-bed facility, with cots installed in every nook, crevice, and cranny. Nurses and doctors had so exhausted themselves caring for the sick that many also now lay ill or dying, having failed, as one observer put it, to "buck the game." Everywhere Welch and Vaughan looked there were men coughing up blood. In many instances, crimson fluids poured from nostrils and ears. Even eight years later the images were still etched in Vaughan's memory. "I see hundreds of young, stalwart men in the uniform of their country coming into the wards of the hospital in groups of ten or more," he wrote in 1926. "They are placed on the cots until every bed is full and yet others crowd in. The faces soon wear a bluish cast; a distressing cough brings up the bloodstained sputum. In the morning the dead bodies are stacked about the morgue like cord wood . . . such are the grewsome [sic] pictures exhibited by the revolving memory cylinders in the brain of an old epidemiologist."

The scene that greeted them in the autopsy room, once they had stepped over the cadavers blocking the entrance, was possibly even more gruesome. Before them, on the autopsy table, lay the corpse of a young man. According to Cole, when they tried to move him, bloody fluids poured from his nose. Nevertheless, Welch decided it was imperative to take a closer look at his lungs. What he saw astonished the veteran pathologist. As Cole recalled: "When the chest was opened and the blue swollen lungs were removed and opened, and Dr.

Welch saw the wet, foamy surfaces with real consolidation, he turned and said, 'This must be some new kind of infection or plague' . . . it shocked me to find that the situation, momentarily at least, was too much even for Dr. Welch."

By the end of October one-third of the camp's population, some 15,000 soldiers, had contracted influenza and 787 had died of the pneumonic complications of the disease. Two-thirds of these pneumonias were of the lobar variety. Such pneumonias tended to have a very rapid onset and terminated in either massive pulmonary hemorrhage or pulmonary edema. The devastation was far more extensive than is usually seen in lobar pneumonias, with damage to the epithelial cells that line the respiratory tract but little evidence of bacterial action. The other type was more akin to an acute aggressive bronchopneumonia and was characterized by more localized changes, from which pathogenic bacteria could usually be cultured at autopsy.

The first kind of pneumonia was unlike anything pathologists had observed before in either lobar or bronchopneumonias, fully justifying Welch's description of it as some new kind of plague. But while Welch's intuition may have been correct, he was not yet ready to abandon old certainties. Perhaps it was the fault of his formative years in Leipzig, followed by his battles to get the American medical profession to embrace the new German laboratory methods, that made him reluctant to challenge the conclusions reached by Pfeiffer as to the etiological role of his bacillus, even when his gut instincts as a pathologist told him that this was something both new and terrifying. Or perhaps it was the fact that by now American scientists trained in the same bacteriological techniques were finding *B. influenzae* in influenza patients with similarly gruesome lung pathologies. Foremost among these were William H. Park, the chief of the laboratory division of the New York City Health Department, and his deputy Anna Williams, both highly respected medical researchers. Mindful of the importance of observing "closely and carefully" and "not to be satis-

fied with . . . half proofs," Welch approached Burt Wolbach, the chief
pathologist of Brigham Hospital, Boston, and asked him to conduct
further autopsies to see if all cases of this influenza shared the same
peculiar lung pathology he had seen at Devens. Next he called the
surgeon general's office to give a detailed description of the disease
and urge that "immediate provision be made in every camp for the
rapid expansion of hospital space." The third person he approached
was Oswald Avery at the Rockefeller Institute.

A methodical medical researcher, famous for his austere lifestyle,
Avery lived for the laboratory. Working with Cole, he had already perfected techniques for identifying the four main subtypes of pneumococcus responsible for lobar pneumonia using specific serums. Next
he had gone on to study how efficiently each type killed mice and in
what dosages—experiments that led him to conclude that virulence
was a function of the ability of the polysaccharide capsule of the pneumococcus to resist ingestion by white blood cells, the immune system's first line of defense against invasive bacteria.

One of the challenges of culturing *Bacillus influenzae* is that it is
a fastidious organism that grows only within a very narrow temperature range and which depends heavily on oxygen, meaning it is usually found only on the surface of culture mediums. Because it tends
to grow singly or in pairs, and its colonies are translucent and lacking
in structure, it is also very easy to miss when looking through the
field of an optical microscope. Pfeiffer had realized that a substrate
of hemoglobin greatly facilitated growth of the bacillus and promoted
his blood agar culture as necessary for establishing it (Pfeiffer recommended pigeon's blood; other researchers used rabbit's blood). Once a
bacteriologist had obtained colonies of the bacillus, the next step was
to stain it with an appropriate dye, wash it with alcohol, then stain
it again with a contrasting dye (Gram-positive bacteria retain crystal
violet stains, whereas *B. influenzae* and other Gram-negative bacteria,
such as mycobacteria, require red counterstains). Such stains could

also be applied directly to slides smeared with sputum from influenza cases. However, a more precise and conclusive method was to prepare pure cultures of the bacillus by inoculating mice with sputum from flu patients and then growing the bacteria from fluids taken from the mice and reintroduced to the blood agar media.

Like other researchers, Avery at first found it difficult to grow Pfeiffer's bacillus from the sputum and bronchial expectorations of flu victims, so, to increase his chances, he refined his methods, adding acids to his agar culture medium and substituting defibrinated blood for untreated blood (other researchers heated the blood or filtered and dried it to separate the hemoglobin from the fibrin). Gradually, as Avery perfected his techniques, he was able to find the bacillus more and more frequently, until he was able to tell Welch it was present in twenty-two of thirty dead soldiers examined at Devens. Wolbach's results were even more definitive: he had found the bacillus in every case he examined at Brigham Hospital. That was enough for Welch, Cole, and Vaughan. "It is established that the influenza at Camp Devens is caused by the bacillus of Pfeiffer," they wired the surgeon general on September 27.

IN FACT, influenza is a viral infection. *B. influenza* is merely a fellow traveler. Like other bacteria commonly found in the mouths, throats, and lungs of influenza patients, it is not the primary cause of the disease, though it may play a role in secondary infections. In the fall of 1918 no one knew this, though some researchers had begun to suspect it. Instead, failure to cultivate *B. influenzae* reflected badly on researchers, not the theory of bacterial causation. Indeed, so dominant was the scientific view that influenza was a bacterial infection that, rather than doubt Pfeiffer's claim, scientists chose to doubt their instruments and methods. If the bacillus could not be cultivated on the first attempt, they needed to improve their culture medium, refine their dyes, and try again.

Anomalies are a common occurrence in science. No two experiments are ever exactly alike, but by refining methods and sharing tools and technologies, scientists are broadly able to reproduce each other's observations and findings, thereby arriving at a consensus that this or that interpretation of the world is correct. That is how knowledge emerges and a particular paradigm comes to be adopted. However, there is no such thing as absolute certainty in science. Paradigms are constantly being refined by new observations and, if enough anomalies are found, faith in the paradigm may be undermined and a new one may come to supplant it. Indeed, the best scientists welcome anomalies and uncertainty, as this is the way science progresses.

When Pfeiffer first advanced his claim for the etiological role of his bacillus, the science of bacteriology and the germ-theory paradigm (one germ, one disease) was in the ascendancy. With the invention of improved achromatic lenses and better culture-staining techniques, by the late 1880s Robert Koch and Louis Pasteur had brought a series of hitherto hard-to-detect germs into view. These included not only such landmark bacteria as the bacilli of fowl cholera and tuberculosis, but streptococcus and staphylococcus. In short order, their discoveries paved the way for the development of serums and bacterial vaccines against diseases such as cholera, typhoid, and plague, and by the eve of World War I, Avery and Cole were using the same methods to develop vaccines for pneumococcal pneumonias.

When Pfeiffer made his announcement in 1892, it raised hopes that it would not be long before bacteriology had also delivered a vaccine for influenza. But from the beginning, Pfeiffer's claim was dogged by doubts and anomalous observations. The first problem was that Pfeiffer had failed to find *B. influenzae* in the majority of clinical cases he had examined in Berlin during the Russian influenza epidemic. Second, as noted previously, he had been unable to reproduce the disease in monkeys inoculated with pure cultures of the bacillus (Pfeiffer does not specify what type of monkey he used, but his failure may have been because many monkeys are a poor refractory species for human influenzas). Soon afterwards, Edward Klein, a Vienna-trained histologist and author of the leading British textbook on bacteriology, succeeded in isolating the bacillus from a series of patients admitted to hospitals in London during the same epidemic of Russian flu. However, Klein also noted finding "crowds" of other bacteria in sputum cultures and observed that as the condition of influenza patients improved, it became progressively more difficult to find Pfeiffer's bacillus in the colonies on the agar plating medium used to grow bacteria. Finally, Klein noted that *B. influenzae* had also been isolated from patients suffering diseases *other than* influenza.

After 1892, the Russian influenza epidemic abated and it was no longer possible to conduct bacteriological exams of influenza patients. Now and then there would be a resurgence of Russian flu, however, and investigators would attempt to culture the bacillus from the sputum and lung secretions of convalescents. Sometimes these efforts succeeded, but just as often they did not. For instance, in 1906 David J. Davis, from the Memorial Institute for Infectious Disease in Chicago, reported being able to isolate the bacillus in only three of seventeen cases of influenza. By contrast he had found the bacillus in all but five of sixty-one cases of whooping cough. The following year, W. D'Este Emery, clinical pathologist at King's College London, noted that *B. infuenzae* grew more readily in culture in the presence of other respiratory bacteria and seemed to be more virulent for animals in the presence of killed streptococci, leading him to speculate that Pfeiffer's bacillus might, for the most part, be a "harmless saprophyte" and that it required other respiratory pathogens to make it pathogenic.

With the emergence of Spanish flu in 1918, researchers were able to resume their investigations. Again, the results were mixed, and again the anomalies cast doubt on Pfeiffer's claim. By the summer, concerns had reached such a pitch that a special meeting was convened at the Munich Medical Union. Summarizing the debate, *The Lancet* wrote that "Pfeiffer's bacillus has been found but exceptionally," and that if any bacteria had a claim to be the cause of influenza it should be the far more common streptococci and pneumococci. Britain's Royal College of Physicians concurred, arguing that there was "insufficient evidence" for Pfeiffer's claim, though it was happy to allow that the bacillus played an important secondary role in fatal respiratory complications of influenza. In other words, the etiological role of B. influenzae might be open to question, but the bacterial paradigm was not. However, this paradigm was now facing a serious challenge from another quarter.

If Koch was the German father of bacteriology, then Louis Pasteur was its French parent or, as one writer puts it, microbiology's "lynchpin." In his first biological paper, published in 1857 at the age of 35, Pasteur, then a relatively unknown French chemist working in Lille, boldly formulated what he called the germ theory of fermentation—namely, that each particular type of fermentation is caused by a specific kind of microbe. In the same paper he suggested that this theory could be generalized into a specific microbial etiology of disease and, later, a general biological principle captured by his phrase, "Life is the germ, and the germ is life." However, in his own lifetime Pasteur's fame rested on a famous set of public experiments conducted two decades later, in which he isolated the bacteria of anthrax and chicken cholera and, using basic chemical techniques (heat or exposure to oxygen), weakened the microbes to the point where they lost their virulence. Next, he demonstrated that these weakened strains could confer protection to animals challenged with fully virulent versions of the same bacteria. In so doing, Pasteur opened up a whole new branch of microbiology: the study of immunology. Pasteur realized that weak or attenuated microbes stimulated the host (sheep in the case of anthrax; chickens in the case of cholera) to produce substances (antibodies) that protected them against challenge with more virulent, disease-causing microbes. Eight years later, in 1885, Pasteur conducted an even more astounding microbiological experiment by applying the same principles to the rabies virus. Taking the spinal cord from a rabid dog, he injected the diseased material into a rabbit, and, when the rabbit fell ill, repeated the procedure with another rabbit. By passaging the virus in rabbits every few days, he was able to heighten its virulence for rabbits, but reduce its virulence for dogs. Next, he went a stage further and removed the spinal cord of a dead rabbit and dried it for fourteen days. This new attenuated virus no longer caused disease in dogs at all. Instead, it immunized them against challenge with fully virulent rabies. Next, Pasteur staged a daring public demonstration by administering his vaccine to a nine-year-old boy, Joseph Meister, who had been bitten in fourteen places by a rabid dog. Meister made a rapid recovery, prompting banner headlines. Other than smallpox, this was the first successful immunization with a virus vaccine, and within a few months Pasteur was inundated with requests from victims of rabid animal attacks from Smolensk to New Jersey. However, perhaps the most remarkable aspect of Pasteur's breakthrough in retrospect is that he developed the vaccine without being able to see the rabies virus or having much idea what a virus was. The reason is that rabies, like other viruses, is too small to be seen through an optical microscope (it measures 150 nanometers, or 0.15 micrometers, and requires magnifications ten thousand times greater than were available in Pasteur's day). But although Pasteur could not visualize the virus or cultivate it in the laboratory, he could intuit its existence by excluding microbes that he could grow and see, i.e., bacteria. Indeed, in 1892, the same year that Pfeiffer had claimed that a bacillus was the cause of influenza, the Russian botanist Dmitry Ivanovski had shown that tobacco mosaic disease was caused by an unseen agent that passed through porcelain filters with pores too small to admit bacteria. By the turn of the century, these filters, known as Chamberland filters after their inventor Charles Chamberland, were being manufactured and used in research laboratories in Europe and elsewhere, leading to the identification of a variety of "filter passing" agents, including the agents of foot and mouth disease of cattle, bovine pleuropneumonia, rabbit myxomatosis, and African horse sickness. Then, in 1902, a commission headed by US Army Surgeon Walter Reed identified the first filter-passing human disease, yellow fever. At the Pasteur Institute in Paris, these agents were referred to as *"virus filtrants"*—"filter-passing viruses."

After his death in 1885, Pasteur's disciples, such as Emile Roux and Roux's star pupil Charles Nicolle, continued these investigations. Dividing his time between biomedical research and administrative duties—it was Roux who created the Pasteur Institute—by 1902 Roux had identified ten diseases that he believed were due to filter-passing viruses. The same year, he persuaded Nicolle to join the Pasteur Institute in Tunis. Though greatly attracted by literature, Nicolle had bowed to the wish of his physician father to study medicine, but while practicing in Rouen had suffered a hearing loss that prevented him from effectively using a stethoscope—an accident that may have persuaded him to concentrate on bacteriology instead and accept the position in North Africa. Nicolle quickly showed himself worthy of Roux's faith, and on arriving in Tunis launched a study of epidemic typhus. At the time, most doctors thought typhus, which tended to decimate armies at times of war and was a particular problem in prisons and other closed institutions, was a disease of filth and squalor. No one realized typhus was actually transmitted by the body louse (*Pediculus humanis corporis*), which infested unlaundered clothing, or that the agent was a tiny intracellular organism belonging to the *Rickettsia* family—the same family responsible for the tick-borne disease, Rocky Mountain spotted fever. Nicolle began by injecting guinea pigs with blood from patients with typhus, showing that, although they did not develop the disease, the inoculations resulted in transient fevers—evidence that they were subclinically, or as Nicole put it, "inapparently" infected by something in the blood. However, the crucial observation came when he was observing typhus patients entering the Sadiki Hospital in Tunis and realized that they ceased to be infectious as soon as their clothing was removed and they were bathed and dressed in hospital uniforms. Suspecting that lice, not dirt, was the cause, Nicolle requested a chimpanzee from Roux and injected the chimp with blood from a typhus patient. When the chimp developed fever and skin eruptions, he injected its blood into a macaque monkey, and when the macaque also fell ill he allowed lice to feed on it. In this way, he was able to transfer the infection to other macaques and, eventually, a chimp. In September 1909, he communicated his finding that lice were the carriers of typhus to the French Academy of Sciences—a discovery for which in 1928 he was awarded the Nobel Prize.

Although Nicolle's efforts to develop a vaccine for typhus would be unsuccessful (this would be left to others), it was only natural that when the influenza epidemic struck he would want to study it using similar methods. There is no evidence that Nicolle had worked on influenza before or had tried to culture its putative bacillus, but by the summer of 1918 French bacteriologists raised in the Pasteurian tradition were finding it increasingly difficult to isolate Pfeiffer's organism and were becoming increasingly skeptical of the German's claims. Instead, Nicolle and his assistant, Charles Lebailly, began to suspect that, like the microbe of yellow fever, influenza might be a filter-passer.

By late August the flu had reached Tunis and there were signs of *la grippe* everywhere. Whether this was an extension of the same flu that had visited Europe in the spring and early part of the summer or a different strain, such as the more virulent strain seen at Devens in the fall of 1918, is difficult to say. The point is that rather than trying to cultivate the bacillus, Nicolle decided to use the same method he had used with typhus. Accordingly, in late August he and Lebailly requested more test animals and began monitoring patients with flu. Chimpanzees were now impossible to obtain, so once again Nicolle settled on macaques, a fortunate choice as it turned out. Nicolle and

Lebailly then looked for a household afflicted by the epidemic to be sure that they were examining a definitive case of *la grippe*, and not some other disease. The patient they selected was a forty-four-year-old man, identified only as "M.M.," who had fallen ill on August 24, together with his daughters. Six days later, M.M. was displaying classic symptoms of influenza—nasopharyngitis, a violent headache, and fever—and Nicolle and Lebailly drew some blood. The following day, September 1, they also collected bronchial expectorations. At this point, Nicolle and Lebailly had no idea if it was possible to transmit flu to a monkey or if the organism responsible for the disease was to be found in human blood, sputum, or other bodily fluids. However, while noting that M.M.'s sputum contained "diverse" bacteria, including *B. influenzae*, they observed that the bacillus was present in "minimal" amounts and did not attempt to prepare pure cultures of the bacillus. Instead, they removed *B.influenzae* and other bacteria from M.M.'s bronchial expectorations using a Chamberland filter and injected the filtrate directly into the eyes and nose of a Chinese bonnet monkey (*Macacus sinicus*). At the same time, they administered the filtrate to two human volunteers, a twenty-two-year-old who was inoculated under the skin, and a thirty-year-old who received the filtrate intravenously. Six days later, both the macaque and the first volunteer came down with symptoms highly suggestive of flu—the monkey developed a fever and marked depression with loss of appetite, while the twenty-two-year-old experienced rapid onset of fever, accompanied by a runny nose, headache, and generalized body aches. As no one else in the first volunteer's living quarters developed influenza at the same time, Nicolle and Lebailly reasoned that the person *had* contracted flu from the filtrate. However, the second volunteer showed no signs of illness, even after fifteen days. Nicolle and Lebailly also attempted to infect other macaques by inoculating them with blood from M.M., but without success (the injections were given in either the monkeys' peritoneal cavities or their brains). Using blood from the macaque, they also inoculated a third volunteer who had developed apparent symptoms of influenza, but this also proved unsuccessful. Finally, on September 15 they repeated the first experiment with a long-tailed macaque (*Macacus cynomologus*) and a fourth volunteer. This time the filtered expectorations resulted in only a slight rise in temperature in the monkey and induced mild symptoms of flu in the volunteer.

By today's standards the experiments were hardly ideal—for instance, Nicolle and Lebailly did not use other monkeys or humans as controls (presumably because macaques were in short supply), nor do they appear to have been "blinded" from their subjects, as would be required today. Moreover, they did not investigate the pathogenic effect of filtered sputum from *noninfluenza* cases, nor were they able to conduct passage experiments, as Pasteur had done with rabies in rabbits, to manipulate the virulence of the organism and reproduce the disease through several generations. Nevertheless, Nicolle and Lebailly concluded that the bronchial expectorations of influenza patients were virulent and that both the bonnet monkey and the long-tailed macaque were susceptible to subcutaneous inoculation with the filtered fluids. Flu therefore was an *"organisme filtrant"*—a filtered organism. They further concluded that the filtered virus had "reproduced the disease" in the two people inoculated subcutaneously.

Nicolle and Lebailly's paper detailing their findings was read by Roux before the French Academy of Sciences in Paris on September 21. In other words, the day before Welch arrived at Devens and witnessed the carnage sweeping the camp. Ordinarily, such an announcement before a respected scientific body would make other researchers around the world sit up and take notice. But the world was in the midst of war and Welch and his colleagues had more pressing concerns. Besides, even if reports of Nicolle and Lebailly's study had reached the surgeon general's office in Washington, DC in time and the news had been communicated to Welch—and there is no evidence that at this stage it was—it is unlikely that he would have given it particular credence. After all, Nicolle and Lebailly's investigations could hardly be considered conclusive. Moreover, before accepting their findings, Welch would have wanted other researchers—preferably American ones—to duplicate their experiments. The ideal place to do this was at the Rockefeller Institute, now an auxiliary laboratory of the US Army, or at nearby naval research laboratories in Boston and Rhode Island. The bacteriological paradigm of influenza could not be overturned on the basis of just a few experiments conducted in North Africa thousands of miles from the main theaters of war and the world's preeminent medical research institutions.

Today, we know that Nicolle and Lebailly's supposition was correct. Influenza *is* a virus. To be precise, it is composed of eight slender strands of ribonucleic acid (RNA)—by contrast the building blocks of human and other mammalian cells are comprised of double-stranded helix spirals of deoxyribonucleic acid (DNA). However, Nicolle and Lebailly were almost certainly not justified in reaching that conclusion based on their experiments. First, while it is possible they could have infected the human volunteers with influenza if they had dripped the filtrate directly into their noses, it is extremely unlikely they could have done so by injecting the filtrate under the skin. That is not to say that the volunteers did not have influenza, only that they probably did not get it the way that Nicolle and Lebailly thought they did. Second, although it is possible to infect a range of Old World monkeys with human flus (squirrel monkeys are particularly susceptible), macaques are a poor refractory species for human influenza and rarely develop visible respiratory symptoms or lung damage. It is also very difficult to get them to "take" the disease by dripping filtrate into their noses or by exposing them to aerosols containing the virus—indeed, in studies conducted in monkeys since 1918 researchers have reported far greater success with intravenous inoculations of the virus, somewhat ironic given Nicolle and Lebailly's reported failure in this respect.

To be fair, in the absence of a reliable animal model for human influenza and a means of propagating the virus in living cells, in 1918 no researcher stood much chance of demonstrating that influenza was a virus. That only became possible after 1933, when a team of British researchers studying canine distemper demonstrated that ferrets were highly sensitive to influenza and could be inoculated simply by introducing filtered sputum into their nasal passages. When, soon after, one of the ferrets sneezed on a scientist who was handling it and the scientist went on to develop flu, the viral etiology of flu was considered proven. This was followed in 1934 by the discovery that influenza viruses could be cultivated in chick egg embryos, freeing researchers from the need to collect samples from patients during an outbreak or forcing them to abandon their research when epidemics ended and the supply of flu patients dried up. With chick embryo cultivation, the virus could now be propagated continuously in the laboratory, and scientists could be sure that they were performing experiments with the same strain of virus, something that had not been possible in 1918. By passaging flu viruses through embryonated hen's eggs, scientists could also attenuate the viruses and manufacture vaccines, thereby providing protection against whichever type of flu happened to be circulating that season.*

UNLIKE AIDS AND SMALLPOX, influenza is not a particularly disfiguring disease; for the most part, it does not leave visible marks or scars on the body. Nor does it cause victims to retch black fluids from their stomachs as yellow fever does, or induce uncontrollable diarrhea as cholera does. But for those who witnessed the disturbing cyanotic end stages of the disease, when victims' lungs were compromised by pneumonia and their cheeks and lips turned blue then dark purple, Spanish flu was shocking to behold. This was not only the case at Devens

---

* Chick egg embryo cultivation is still the principal means of making flu vaccines.

and other US Army camps, but on the transatlantic troopships that conveyed American soldiers to Europe. On the *Leviathan*, a massive transport that set sail from New York at the end of September, eyewitnesses described having to step through "pools of blood from severe nasal hemorrhages." At first men were confined to steel cabins below deck in the hope of containing the infection, but within days of leaving New York so many were ill and the stench below decks was so overpowering that they were brought outside to breathe the sea air. In an era before antibiotics, and with no vaccine, doctors were powerless to heal the afflicted. Instead, they distributed fresh fruit and water. Sadly, like the bloody discharges, these also soon ended up on the floor, so that the decks became "wet and slippery, [with the] groans and cries of the terrified added to the confusion of the applicants clamoring for treatment." By the time the *Leviathan* arrived at Brest on October 8, some 2,000 soldiers were ill and eighty had died, the majority of their bodies having been disposed of at sea.

New Yorkers were unaware of the dreadful scenes on the *Leviathan*. When the vessel set sail, most New Yorkers still thought of Spanish influenza as an exotic foreign disease. Public health officials, keen to contribute to the war effort, colluded in the deception, downplaying the flu's impact on American servicemen even as they talked up the toll it was exacting on German troops. "You haven't heard of our doughboys getting it, have you?" queried New York's Commissioner of Health Royal S. Copeland. "You bet you haven't, and you won't." Slowly but surely, however, the virus was swimming closer to shore, conveyed in the bodies of the passengers and crew of returning troopships and commercial liners. And all the while, as it passaged through more and more bodies, it was growing in virulence. The result was that when it made landfall soldiers would not be the only casualties.

It is difficult to say how and where the second wave broke. Perhaps the fall outbreak began at Commonwealth Pier, in Boston, before spreading to Ayer and other towns in Massachusetts. Or perhaps there were several simultaneous introductions of the virus. New York, for instance, saw a marked increase in influenza deaths, particularly in middle age groups, in February–April 1918, though the first cases in the second wave were associated with passengers alighting from a Norwegian steamer in the middle of August. By the end of September, cases in New York were running at eight hundred a day, and Copeland took the unusual step of ordering quarantines (wealthy patients were allowed to remain in their homes, but those living in boarding houses or tenements were removed to city hospitals where they were kept under strict observation). Quarantines were something new and unprecedented for influenza—before the war, flu had not even been a notifiable disease—and New Yorkers could not help but be reminded of the polio epidemic two years earlier. Then, officials had gone door-to-door rounding up children with symptoms of "infantile paralysis," spreading terror in neighborhoods like Brooklyn where recent Italian immigrants were suspected of harboring the disease. However, the Spanish flu was as likely to visit a Park Avenue brownstone as a Brooklyn tenement, and as each day brought new reports of sickness, the city grew increasingly uneasy. Copeland tried to reassure New Yorkers by explaining that influenza was only communicable "in the coughing and sneezing of one who actually has influenza," not from someone living in the same household as someone stricken with flu but who did not show symptoms. He also insisted that a vaccine was imminent. He was referring to the efforts by scientists like Park and Williams at the New York public health laboratory who were experimenting with vaccines using mixed strains of B. influenzae. By the middle of October, Park was reporting that animals immunized with a heat-killed vaccine made from these bacterial cocktails showed specific antibodies against the bacillus. Scientists at Tufts Medical School in Boston and the University of Pittsburgh's medical school were reporting similar progress with their own version of heat-killed bacterial vaccines. But while Park was having more success culturing *B. influenzae* and getting it to agglutinate to antibodies in serum, privately he was beginning to worry that the results might be a reflection of improved culture techniques rather than proof of the bacillus's etiological role. "There is of course the possibility that some unknown filterable virus may be the starting point," he wired a colleague. In spite of these misgivings, Park's vaccine was eventually released to the military. It was also used to immunize 275,000 employees of the US Steel Company. There is no evidence that these primitive vaccines and serums had any effect on influenza whatsoever.

By October 6, more than 2,000 people a day in New York were being quarantined and the panic was palpable. From several districts came reports that patients were holding nurses captive in their homes because they were so frightened. Then nurses and doctors also starting falling sick. By now the flu had reached San Francisco and was also raging in cities in the Midwest and South. The flu erupted in Chicago in mid-September, most likely introduced by sailors from the nearby Great Lakes Naval Station. With a capacity for 45,000 men, the station was the largest naval training facility in the world, and, like Devens, a breeding ground for respiratory disease. As flu and pneumonia gripped Chicago, citizens were advised to avoid crowds and other public gatherings and to cover their mouths when sneezing. The most visible signs of the contagion were the gauze face masks worn by policemen and tram attendants. The trend quickly caught on, prompting a prominent Illinois physician to warn that homemade masks were inadequate because they were "made from gauze with meshes too large to catch and strain out the bacilli from the fine spray issuing from the mouths of victims." This was of special concern in hospitals and other confined spaces as the spray was thought to be infectious at distances of up to twenty feet. Instead, he persuaded the *Chicago Herald Examiner* to publish a cut-out-and-keep guide on its front page for the proper procedure for making a gauze mask with a narrow mesh. Unfortunately, these masks made little difference as

influenza virus particles are many times smaller than the smallest
bacteria, and by mid-October Chicago was already reporting 40,000
cases. The hardest hit city of all, however, was Philadelphia.

By 1918 Philadelphia had grown considerably since its Quaker
beginnings as the capital of the Pennsylvania colony and the place
where the founding fathers signed the Declaration of Independence.
Ringed by steel mills and with its huge shipyards overlooking the Del-
aware River, Philadelphia was an industrial powerhouse. The needs of
war (naval vessels, aircraft, munitions) brought tens of thousands of
additional workers flocking to the city, and as its population swelled
to nearly two million, so living conditions in Philadelphia became
increasingly intolerable. In cramped rooming houses and overcrowded
tenements, the virus found ample fodder and steadily increased in
virulence, killing people rapidly and indiscriminately. At a time when
authorities in other cities were advising people to avoid large public
gatherings, the epidemic was almost certainly exacerbated by the decision of Philadelphia's mayor to proceed with a Liberty Loan Drive on
September 28. The drive brought thousands of people crowding into
the downtown area, and within two weeks Philadelphia had recorded
more than 2,600 flu deaths. By the third week of October deaths had
soared to over 4,500. As bodies piled up in morgues for lack of under-
takers, the stench became overpowering and the city resorted to dig-
ging mass graves—something that had not been seen since the yellow
fever epidemics of the late eighteenth century. The sight of rotting
bodies became so commonplace that adults made little effort to shield
children from the horrors. The fear of influenza was now palpable, and
with fear came panic. But this panic was not the press' fault. "Panic
is the worst thing that can happen to an individual or a community,"
warned the *Philadelphia Inquirer* in an editorial at the height of the fall
wave. "Panic is exaggerated fear and fear is the most deadly word in
any language." The remedy, it suggested, was to expel fearful thoughts
by an act of will. "Do not dwell on the influenza. Do not even discuss

it. . . . Terror is a big ally of the influenza." But once seen, the sight of a cyanotic, influenza-ridden body was not easily forgotten, either in Philadelphia or other places the flu visited. The sight of "big strong men, heliotrope blue and breathing 50 to the minute" was unforgettable, observed Dr. Herbert French, a pathologist based at Guy's Hospital in London and a physician to Her Majesty's Household. But the worst case by far was the type that became "totally unconscious hours or even days before the end, restless in his coma, with head thrown back, mouth half open, a ghastly sallow pallor of the cyanosed face, purple lips and ears." It was "a dreadful sight," he concluded.

THE 1918 INFLUENZA pandemic was a shot heard around the world. The scenes described by French were not confined only to London and other large European and American cities but were the same everywhere. In Cape Town, observed one eyewitness, the fall wave "made orphans of between two to three thousand children." One such orphan who was co-opted into burial duties reported: "I carry the coffin, holding my nose . . . no longer were church bells tolling for the dead . . . there was no sexton to ring the bells." It was the same in Bombay (Mumbai), where the disease arrived courtesy of a container ship in May. Deaths peaked in the first week of October, the same time as Boston. By the end of the year, the flu had killed an estimated one million people in this populous Indian city. All told, the pandemic claimed the lives of 18.5 million people across the Indian subcontinent, according to the latest estimates, and perhaps as many as 100 million worldwide. With the exception of Australia, where strict maritime quarantines delayed the onset of flu until the winter of 1919, virtually the entire globe suffered the pandemic at the same time. Only American Samoa, St. Helena, and a handful of islands in the South Atlantic escaped the plague. It was truly a shared global disaster.

It is difficult to imagine deaths of this order of magnitude, much less process them. The scale is too vast. "When one has fought a war, one hardly knows any more what a dead person is," remarks Camus. "And if a dead man has no significance unless one has seen him dead, a hundred million bodies spread through history are just a mist drifting through the imagination." However, if there is little point in trying to imagine death on this scale, there is much to be gained from examining variations in mortality rates observed in different geographical locations and ecological and immunological settings. When influenza reached New Zealand, for instance, the local Maori population died at seven times the rate of British settlers. Similarly wide variations in mortality rates were observed between indigenous and European-descended peoples in Fiji and other South Pacific islands (one of the most striking discrepancies was observed in Guam, where the pandemic killed 5 percent of the local population but just one sailor at the US naval base on the island). While the case fatality rate for "white" South Africans was 2.6 percent, for "blacks, Indians, and Coloureds" it was nearly 6 percent. For those who toiled underground in the Kimberley diamond mines the mortality rate was even worse—22 percent. Similar variations were observed at Devens and other large army training camps, with recent arrivals suffering far worse clinical outcomes than men of a similar age who had been at the camps for four months or longer. On the AEF transports, sailors permanently assigned to the ships fared far better than soldiers who had just embarked, even though both were attacked by influenza in more or less equal numbers.

But perhaps the most striking aspect of the Spanish flu pandemic was the mortality pattern observed in young adults. In a normal flu season, curves of mortality by age at death are typically U-shaped, reflecting high mortality in the very young (children under three) and the elderly (seventy-five and over), with low mortality at all ages in between. This is because infants and the aged tend to be those with the weakest immune systems. By contrast, the 1918–1919 pandemic and the succeeding winter recurrences in 1919 and 1920 produced a W-shaped curve, with a third mortality peak in adults aged 20–40 years. Moreover, adults in these age ranges were responsible for half the total influenza deaths, including the majority of excess respiratory deaths. This abnormal mortality pattern was observed both in cities and rural areas, in major European metropolises and distant outposts of empire. In other words, it was the same everywhere.

Why this should have been the case has never been satisfactorily explained. Nor, despite the advances in influenza virology and immunology and a better understanding of the pathophysiology of flu, are scientists today in a much better position to say whether the Spanish flu pandemic was a one-off occurrence—a never-to-be-repeated epidemiological disaster—or whether it could happen again. By reviewing what has been learned about the 1918 virus, and the likely identity of previous pandemic viruses, it is possible to rule out some hypotheses and rule others in. However, perhaps the biggest clue to the epidemiological patterns and unusual lung pathologies observed in 1918 comes from the ecology of large army camps and the contemporary accounts of medics who observed the ravages wrought by influenza in them at first hand.

INFLUENZA, WE NOW KNOW, is a member of the family *Orthomyxoviridae*, and comes in three types—A, B, and C—named in the order of their discovery. Type C rarely causes disease in humans. Type B can cause epidemics, but the course of infection is milder and the spread of the virus tends to be slower. By contrast, type A is associated with explosive spread and high rates of morbidity and mortality, making it the leading cause of epidemics and pandemics. Like all influenza viruses, type A influenzas are RNA viruses and must infect a living cell in order to replicate. Generally, they do this by attacking the epithelial cells that line the respiratory tract from the nose and through the windpipe to the lungs.

Although in 1933 scientists had demonstrated that influenza was a virus that could be transferred from ferrets to man (the breakthrough was made by a team headed by Sir Patrick Laidlaw at the Farm Laboratory, in Mill Hill, north London, part of the UK's National Institute for Medical Research), it was not until the 1940s and the invention of the electron microscope that researchers were able to see the influenza virion for the first time. It measured approximately 100 nanometers (0.10 micrometers), making it slightly smaller than the rabies virus but larger than rhinovirus, the cause of the common cold. Magnified, it resembled nothing so much as the surface of a dandelion bristling with tiny spikes and mushroom-like spines. The spikes are made of a protein called hemagglutinin (HA) that derives its name from its ability to agglutinate to red blood cells. When a person inhales an air droplet containing the virus, it is these spikes that stick to the receptors on the surface of the epithelial cells in the respiratory tract, much as a prickly seed case catches on the fibers of clothing in tall grass. The square-headed mushroom-like protrusions, fewer in number, consist of a powerful enzyme, neuraminidase (NA). It is the combination of these proteins and enzymes that enables the virus to invade epithelial cells and evade the body's immune defenses. These permutations of proteins and enzymes give each virus a signature shape, making for easy classification. In all, scientists have identified sixteen types of hemagglutinin and nine types of neuraminidase in mammals and birds (besides ferrets, type A flu viruses commonly infect pigs, whales, seals, horses, and wild waterfowl), but so far only three types of each have been found to readily infect humans. These are labeled H_1, H_2, and H_3, and N_1 and N_2, respectively. The Spanish flu is an H_1N_1.

Unlike DNA, RNA does not possess an accurate proofreading mechanism. During replication, when the virus invades and colonizes animal cells, the RNA makes small copying errors, resulting in genetic mutations to the H and N molecules on its surface. In the Darwinian world of the virus, some of these copies can confer a competitive advantage, allowing the viruses to escape the antibodies designed to neutralize them and enabling them to spread more efficiently via coughs and sneezes to the wider environment ready to infect the next person. This process of gradual mutation is known as "antigenic drift." Type A viruses can also spontaneously "swap" or exchange genetic material. This process is typically thought to occur in intermediary hosts such as pigs, which can be infected with swine and human type A strains simultaneously, and is known as "antigenic shift." In this case, the result is the emergence of a completely new subtype that codes for proteins that may be new to the immune system and for which human populations may possess few or no antibodies. It is these strains that historically have been the cause of pandemics. However, it is thought that the virus responsible for the 1918 pandemic may have emerged in yet another way.

In the 1990s scientists at the Armed Forces Institute of Pathology in Bethesda, Maryland, led by molecular pathologist Jeffery Taubenberger, succeeded in retrieving fragments of the Spanish flu virus from lung autopsy specimens stored in the institute's archives. Further genetic viral material came from a woman who had died of influenza in 1918 in Alaska and had been buried in permafrost, which preserved her lungs from decay. Using this material, Taubenberger's group was eventually able to sequence the virus's entire genome. Published in 2005, the results came as something of a surprise because none of the eight genes came from a strain that had previously infected humans, as one would have expected if the Spanish flu had been the result of antigenic shift. Furthermore, large portions of the genetic code matched sequences only found in wild birds. This suggested that the virus may have begun as a bird-adapted strain that, with just a handful of mutations, made the leap to humans. Alternatively, the pandemic strain may have begun life as an H1 which reassorted with an avian virus shortly before 1918. By zoos, it was recognized that mallards and teals were an important reservoir of avian influenza viruses in the wild, and the idea that birds might be the source of novel genes in pandemic viruses was gaining currency. Taubenberger's sequencing studies also coincided with growing concern about an avian virus that was then infecting chicken flocks across Southeast Asia. The virus, known as H5N1, had first emerged in Hong Kong in 1997, where it infected eighteen people and caused six deaths, before reemerging for a second time in 2002. Since then the virus had spread from Asia to Europe and Africa, sparking hundreds of human cases and forcing authorities to cull millions of chickens. Alarmingly, the H5N1 virus was able to replicate in the human respiratory tract, and the mortality rate averaged 60 percent. However, it did not transmit easily from person to person. Nevertheless, its emergence demonstrated that people could be directly infected with a wholly avian influenza virus, meaning it was no longer necessary to invoke pigs as intermediary hosts in the generation of pandemic strains. Theoretically, such reassortments, or mixing, of avian and mammalian flu strains could also occur in humans. The question was, could something like this have happened in 1918? The short answer is that no one knows, but the possibility cannot be ruled out.

The precise genetic identities of pandemic strains prior to 1900 are lost to history, but in the twentieth century there have been three major shifts. The first was the H1N1 Spanish flu virus that emerged in 1918, or possibly a little earlier (by comparing older and more recent strains of the virus and running molecular clocks backward in time, evolutionary biologists suggest the virus may have acquired its avian genes somewhere between 1913 and 1917). This was the prevailing strain until 1957, when it was replaced by a new viral strain, typed H2N2. Known as the "Asian flu," the H2N2 seems to have been generated by a reassortment of descendants of the 1918 virus with an avian influenza strain derived from Eurasian wild waterfowl. It spread rapidly around the globe, displacing descendants of H1N1 Spanish flu and killing an estimated two million people. In 1968 there was a third shift, when an

H3N2 suddenly emerged in Hong Kong, also apparently as a result of the acquisition of novel proteins from Eurasian wild waterfowl. Known, unsurprisingly, as the "Hong Kong" flu, this virus is estimated to have killed one million people globally, and at the time of writing remains the leading cause of morbidity and mortality from influenza.

To complete the picture of pandemic viruses in the modern period, we also need to include the Russian flu. Like the 1918 Spanish flu, this was a true worldwide pandemic. Originating in the Eurasian "steppes"—a vast expanse of grassland that encompassed parts of Russia plus Tsarist-controlled Uzbekistan and Kazakhstan—it spread rapidly along international rail and shipping routes and is conservatively thought to have killed one million in the period between 1889 and 1892. Unfortunately, scientists have been unable to recover fragments of the virus, so its precise genetic identity is unknown. However, serology tests on elderly people who were examined for antibodies at the time of the 1968 Hong Kong flu suggest that, like that virus, it was caused by an H3. This may be an important clue, as those most at risk of dying in 1918 were born in or around 1890, meaning they belonged to a birth cohort whose first exposure to a flu virus would almost certainly have been to the Russian flu. We will return to this in a moment, but first it is necessary to consider the nature of the pneumonias that killed people in 1918.

As noted earlier, broadly speaking these pneumonias can be divided into two types—lobar and bronchial. However, it is also important to note that in a previrological era, these distinctions rested on clinical observations and histological examinations of lung tissue and that the two types were often closely related, with the clinical-pathological syndromes sometimes overlapping. The most common type by far appears to have been an acute aggressive bronchopneumonia. In this type, pathological changes were most obvious in the bronchi, and pathogenic bacteria could usually be cultured at autopsy from different parts of the lung. Close to 90 percent of the pneumonias fell into this category. In the second type, the outstanding features were pulmonary hemorrhage and edema with extensive damage to one or more of the lobes, and pathogenic bacteria were less frequently or rarely recovered. In this type, the infection appears to have triggered an acute inflammation of the pulmonary alveoli resulting in cell death (necrosis) and the deposit of damaged cells and fluids in the alveolar air spaces—the microscopic sacs that absorb oxygen in the lung. These features were found whenever victims died within a few days of the onset of illness, as well as in 70 percent of cases in which pneumonia developed after influenza. And they were nearly always found in deaths involving healthy young soldiers or civilians. However, it must be reiterated that this type accounted for only a small percentage of deaths overall. The later-onset bronchopneumonias and mixed infections, in which bacteria could be readily cultured after death, were the ones encountered most frequently. Indeed, it is these bacterial fellow travelers of flu—or what pathologists at the time called "secondary invaders"—that many experts believe best explain the majority of deaths seen at camps like Devens and the variations in mortality observed between recruits of the same age from rural and urban areas.

It is perhaps also worth remarking that as doubts about the etiological role of B. influenzae grew, so pathologists took care to distinguish between lung lesions attributable to commensal bacteria and those due to the presumed, though as yet unproven, virus of the epidemic. By the mid-1920s, this was a view that Welch was also coming to endorse. Addressing a meeting of public health officials in Boston in 1926, Welch said that the idea that influenza was due to an "unknown virus" had much to recommend it, and he now thought that "when there was a lesion of the lung . . . it was attributable to the virus, the real influenza virus, not general respiratory manifestations." He had also been struck by the "crowding together" of soldiers at the base hospital at Devens, an occurrence that he thought increased patients' risk of exposure to other organisms and was "largely responsible for the enormous extent of the disease."

Unlike in 1918, today it is possible to study the virus in the laboratory using a process called reverse genetics. Beginning in 2005, this is exactly what scientists have done, reassembling the virus in Biosafety Level Four facilities and then challenging mice and other test animals. The resurrected virus kills mice in three to five days and causes a severe lung inflammation reminiscent of the lesions reported by doctors in 1918. It also replicates very efficiently in bronchial epithelial cells. Indeed, so striking is the virulence of the 1918 virus in animal models that some virologists argue that infection with the virus alone could have triggered the rapid onset pneumonias and symptoms of cyanosis described by pathologists in 1918 and that it is unnecessary to invoke secondary bacterial invaders. One suggestion is that the pneumonias and symptoms of cyanosis may have been due to an overly exuberant immune response involving the release of proinflammatory cells called cytokines. This phenomenon—known as a "cytokine storm"—was implicated in the deaths from Acute Respiratory Distress Syndrome (ARDS) that followed the H5N1 bird flu outbreaks in Southeast Asia in the early 2000s, and has also been observed with other epidemic viruses such as SARS.

Whether or not these pneumonias were primarily viral or bacterial, or a mixture of both, does not answer the question why the Spanish flu proved so deadly to young adults in the prime of life, however. Here, present-day science has several hypotheses but no good answers. One suggestion is that older age groups enjoyed greater protection because they had previously been exposed to a similar virus. This fits with serological evidence suggesting that people born between 1830 and 1889 were also exposed to an H1. It was only after 1890 that this virus was replaced by a new pandemic virus, the Russian H3. In other words, those aged thirty-eight and over would have already possessed some antibodies to the H1N1 Spanish flu, and in the case of the very elderly—those born in 1834 and who had been infants when they first encountered an H1—this protection would have been considerable.

Another suggestion is that the virus that was to become the Spanish flu (in a scenario where it acquired avian genes around 1915) may have begun life as an H1 that emerged shortly after 1900. This could have been critical for those born in the first years of the twentieth century and who would have been eighteen or younger at the time the pandemic struck, as it is thought that early life infection with influenza results in an immunological "blind spot." Usually referred to as "original antigenic sin," the idea is that antibodies to the first-encountered flu strain are more readily "recalled" and produced at the expense of new antibodies specific to newer flu strains. It is even possible that through a process known as antibody-dependent enhancement, the older immune response might aid the virus to evade the body's defenses and infect cells more readily. However, while the advantage of such hypotheses is that they help explain why, no matter where the flu struck, the mortality fell most heavily on twenty-to-forty-year-olds, most experts feel that without knowing the precise genetic identity of the 1890 virus and the viruses that came before and after, and the precise immunological profiles of the affected age groups, these hypotheses are somewhat speculative. As David Morens, a medical epidemiologist who works closely with Taubenberger, points out, it is equally possible that the W-shaped mortality pattern could be due to some as yet unidentifiable environmental exposure peculiar to young adults at the time. We just do not know. Indeed, for all that new molecular techniques and a better understanding of the ecology and immunology of flu have brought new insights into the patterns of pandemics, Taubenberger and Morens argue that "we have moved ever further from certainty about the determinants of, and possibilities for pandemic emergence." It is this uncertainty that makes flu—and the 1918 pandemic in particular—such an enigmatic and enduring object of scientific interest and source of anxiety.

But perhaps for the last word on the pandemic we should leave North America and turn to someone who viewed the spreading global morbidity and mortality from the periphery. In 1919, at the age of twenty, Frank Macfarlane Burnet was studying medicine at the University of Melbourne when he suffered an attack of influenza. Thankfully, the illness proved mild. Nevertheless, it left an indelible impression, igniting a lifelong fascination with flu and with what Burnet called "the natural history of infectious disease." In 1931, Burnet arrived at the National Institute for Medical Research in London on a two-year fellowship to study the burgeoning new field of virus diseases. His arrival coincided with the discovery that ferrets could be infected with influenza, and on his return to Melbourne in 1934 he pioneered the technique for growing the virus in chick egg embryos. This would be the first in a series of contributions to influenza research by Burnet—research that would see him investigate variations in virulence between newly isolated and chick-cultivated viruses and lay the ground for future genetic insights into the emergence of pandemics. Intrigued by Nicolle and Lebailly's findings in Tunis in 1918, in 1941 Burnet also conducted a series of trials in macaques, challenging the monkeys with several strains of egg-propagated virus. Although none of the monkeys developed a fever or other signs of illness when infected intranasally, several became ill when Burnet injected the virus directly into their trachea, and at autopsy one showed signs of extensive bronchopneumonia. However, it was the epidemiology of influenza that fascinated Burnet most, and the more he studied the patterns of morbidity and mortality in 1918, the more convinced he became that it was the concentration of recruits from rural and urban districts in overcrowded barracks that held the key to the pandemic's unusual characteristics. Like Welch and the members of the pneumonia commission, Burnet was persuaded that the emergence of Spanish flu was, as he put it, "intimately linked to war conditions," and that it was the immunological profiles of American recruits, followed by their transfer to northern France, where they were able to mix freely with men from other nations, that accounted for the extreme virulence of the virus and the unusual age profile of its victims. "If the early American epidemics supplied the initial spark for the pandemic we can be certain that it was fanned into a flame in Europe," Burnet concluded. But what struck Burnet as possibly even more significant from an immunological point of view was how many people had been *unaffected* by the pandemic. Thus two-thirds of the population had escaped infection altogether, and the overall mortality, as a measure of the total population, had been just 2 percent. While that was twenty-five times higher than in a normal flu season, it was far lower than the mortality rate seen during outbreaks of cholera and pneumonic plague in the nineteenth century, and went some way to explaining why, except for at the height of the killing wave in October, when hospitals had been flooded with pneumonia cases and the deaths had become impossible to ignore, the pandemic had not provoked greater fear and panic. Yes, influenza had briefly presented as "some new kind of plague." But by November 1918 and the declaration of the armistice it was already once more on its way to becoming a perennial seasonal ailment. Unfortunately, that would not be true of other twentieth- and twenty-first-century epidemics caused by similar ecological imbalances and environmental disturbances.

CHAPTER II

PLAGUE IN THE CITY OF ANGELS

"The word 'plague' had just been uttered for the first time."

—ALBERT CAMUS, *The Plague*

O n October 3, 1924, Dr. Giles Porter, a Los Angeles city health officer, was called to the home of a railroad worker in the heart of the Mexican quarter. A few days earlier, Jesus Lajun and his fifteen-year-old daughter, Francisca Concha Lajun, had fallen ill at their apartment at 700 Clara Street, and both were now running high temperatures. Francisca also had a spasmodic, rattling cough, while Jesus had a nasty swelling on his groin. Porter attributed Jesus's swelling to "venereal adenitis" due to syphilis, while Francisca's symptoms of fever and coughing, he thought, were most likely due to influenza. "This child was not considered to be in a serious condition," he recorded in his report. But Porter was wrong and two days later Luciana Samarano, the owner of a nearby boarding house who had been nursing Francisca, became so concerned about the girl's condition that she called an ambulance. Francisca died en route to Los Angeles General Hospital, a pathologist later listing the cause of death as "double pneumonia." For an otherwise healthy teenager to suffer a severe attack of pneumonia was a highly unusual occurrence, but Clara Street was surrounded by brickyards and gas and electrical works, and even in fine weather the air was choked with pollutants.

Taking into account the unpleasant odors emanating from the nearby meatpacking plants, it came as little surprise that Mexicans were the only people prepared to live in the environs of Clara Street or that a young life had been taken prematurely.

Built in 1895 on a vacant plot near the Los Angeles River, Clara Street had originally been an affordable white middle-class neighborhood, but as the city expanded and a land and building boom brought a demand for brick makers and cheap agricultural labor, the Italian residents had moved out and the area had been colonized by Hispanics and migrant workers from south of the border. By 1924 some 2,500 Mexicans were packed into the 307 houses in and around Clara Street, an eight-block area bounded on the east by the Southern Pacific Railroad, on the west by Alameda Street, and on the south by Macy Street. Overcrowding was rife. Many, such as Samarano's home at 742 Clara Street, had been subdivided into "apartments" or transformed into boarding houses in which up to thirty people resided at a time. Other guests bedded down in shacks appended to the rear of the simple clapboard dwellings. People were not the only lodgers. The crawl spaces beneath the floorboards also provided sanctuary for rats and, on occasion, ground squirrels. In short, it was a world away from the Los Angeles described by realtors as the city "of eternal youth—a city without slums."

In the 1920s, Los Angeles had a population of one million and was one of the fastest growing urban centers in the United States. Billed as the "climatic capital of the world," the city was in the midst of a real estate boom as Americans tired of the harsh midwestern winters and the overcrowded conditions in cities in the East flocked to Southern California, attracted by the promise of a new life in a land blessed by oil, palm trees, abundant farmland, and sunshine. Most of these settlers made for the new bedroom communities with names like "Petroleum Gardens" that were springing up on reclaimed desert just beyond the city limits. By contrast, Hispanics tended to congregate in

Macy District—as the Mexican quarter was officially known—or the adjacent Mariana and Belvedere Gardens districts.

By 1924, Los Angeles's Hispanic population totaled around 22,000, and the signs of their labor were everywhere: it was Mexican hands, toiling in the clay pits adjacent to the Los Angeles River, that had fashioned the bricks for the high rises transforming L.A.'s skyline, and it was Mexicans who kept the grocery stores stocked with fresh fruit and vegetables and who scrubbed the floors of the swank downtown hotels. Yet for the city's majority Anglo-Saxon population, these brown-skinned inhabitants of the City of Angels were all but invisible. Sure, there may have been concerns from time to time about the diseases they were presumed to carry, or the demographic implications of the burgeoning Hispanic birthrate, but as Harry Chandler, the owner of the antiunion *Los Angeles Times*, and a prominent Californian landowner and power broker, reassured Congress: Mexicans "do not intermarry like the negro with white people. They don't mingle. They keep to themselves. That is the *safety* of it" (emphasis added).

Seven days after Francisca Lajun's death, her father Jesus also succumbed to the mysterious infection. Then, five days later, Luciana Samarano was admitted to County General, dying on October 19 of "myocarditis" or heart disease (six months' pregnant at the time, Luciana's unborn child died with her). The next casualties were Samarano's husband, Guadalupe, followed by several mourners who had attended Luciana's wake, which, as per Catholic tradition, saw relatives filing past the open casket and kissing the corpse to pay their respects. As with Francisca Lajun, Guadalupe's death was listed as "double pneumonia." By now, several other people who had attended Luciana's wake had also fallen ill with similar symptoms. However, it was only on October 29 that the hospital dispatched its chief resident, Dr. Emil Bogen, to investigate. Bogen's first stop was a house at 343 Carmelita Street in Belvedere Gardens. "In the middle of the room," Bogen recalled, "an old Mexican woman was lying on a large double bed, crying between paroxysms of coughing, while along the wall was a couch on which was seen a Mexican man of about 30 years of age, restless and feverish, but not coughing." Several other people were also present, and one agreed to act as Bogen's interpreter. Bogen was told that the man had fallen sick the day before, that he had a pain along his spine, and that he was running a temperature of 104 degrees. He also had red spots on his chest. The old woman, meanwhile, "had been coughing for the past two days, expectorating a profuse bloody sputum, and had loud, coarse rhonchi."

Bogen arranged for the couple to be transferred to an ambulance, then went with the interpreter to the adjacent house where another man and his wife and daughter were ill with similar symptoms. The wife informed Bogen that she felt better than previously while the daughter "insisted that she was not sick, only a little tired." Within three days, however, both the woman and the girl were in a critical condition at County General, and the woman's husband was dead. Only later did it emerge that he was Guadalupe Samarano's brother, Victor, and that both he and his wife had recently attended the wake at 742 Clara Street. There, Bogen found four desperately sick boys between the ages of four and twelve, the recently orphaned sons of Luciana and Guadalupe. "The four boys were brought to the hospital that same night, and during the following day six more cases were admitted from that neighborhood," he recorded. "Soon after admission they developed signs of a severe pneumonia, with bloody expectoration and marked cyanosis."

Samarano's home would subsequently be labeled the "death house." In all, thirty-three people who had attended Luciana's wake or who were related to the Samaranos or who had lodged at 742 Clara Street would contract plague, and thirty-one would die. The sequence of illnesses was laid out in an official report in which the casualties were listed according to their initials and their relationship to "L.S." or "G.S." After the Samaranos, the next casualty was "J.F.," or Jessie Flores, a family friend and next door neighbor who had nursed Luciana. Then came two of the couple's sons by different marriages, and both Luciana and Guadalupe's mothers. Even the family priest, Father Medardo Brualla, contracted the disease. Brualla had gone to 742 Clara Street on October 26 to administer the last rites to Guadalupe and Jessie, but a few days later he was also expectorating bloody sputum, and by November 2 he was dead.

After Guadalupe's death, unsuspecting health officials had released his body so that his family could pay their respects. Once again, they held the service at 742 Clara Street, and once again, mourners who attended the wake fell ill soon after. By October 30, some twelve people were in critical condition at County General. It was one of these, Horace Gutiérrez, a cousin of Luciana Samarano, who would provide the crucial evidence that would alert health officials to the identity of the pathogen and plunge the Los Angeles Chamber of Commerce and city hall into panic. In his summary, Bogen records that Horace had arrived at the hospital at around the same time as the four Samarano boys, and, shortly after, had developed the same symptoms of pneumonia accompanied by bloody expectorations and cyanosis. As cyanosis had been a signature symptom of the Spanish influenza and the epidemic was still fresh in physicians' memories, the immediate suspicion was flu. In the end, however, the cases were attributed to "epidemic meningitis." Only the hospital's pathologist, Dr. George Maner, thought differently, suggesting that perhaps they were dealing with plague. Later, Maner decided to check his intuition by taking a sputum sample from Gutiérrez and examining it under a microscope. What he saw filled him with dread. Gutiérrez's sputum was packed with tiny rod-shaped bacteria that looked distinctly like the images Maner had seen in textbooks of *Pasteurella pestis*, the bacterium of plague. Unsure of the bacteria's morphology and wanting to get a second opinion, Maner approached his predecessor as chief of pathology at Los Angeles General, a Scotsman by the name of Roy Hammack.

Hammack had previously served in the Philippines, where he had treated several cases of plague, so he had the advantage of having seen the bacillus before. "Beautiful!" he supposedly exclaimed when he espied the familiar rod-shaped bacteria through his microscope. "Beautiful but damned."

⊰⊱

PASTEURELLA PESTIS, or Yersinia pestis to give the bacillus its proper name, is one of the deadliest pathogens known to man. Named for the Swiss bacteriologist, Alexandre Yersin, who isolated the microbe during the third plague pandemic in Hong Kong in 1894, Y. pestis is conservatively thought to have been responsible for 100 million deaths throughout history, perhaps as many as 200 million. Yet for all the horror evoked by the word plague, human infections are only incidental events in the life cycle of the parasite. The bacillus's natural reservoir is wild rodents, such as marmots, ground squirrels, and rats. Transmitted by the bites from infected fleas that live in the rodents' burrows, Y. pestis circulates for the most part harmlessly in these rodent populations. It is only when the relative immunity of rodent populations wanes, and there are sudden die-offs, leaving fleas temporarily homeless, or diseased rodents are brought closer to human habitations, that the existence of the zoonosis becomes visible and there is a risk of transfer of the infection to humans or some other animal host. From the point of view of the parasite and its survival, however, this is not a great strategy, as this "accidental" transfer usually results in the death of its new host, preventing further onward transmission of the bacillus.

The human disease takes three forms: bubonic, septicemic, and pneumonic. The bubonic form occurs when a flea jumps from a rat or some other rodent and bites a human, injecting the plague bacilli under the skin (afterwards, human fleas or body lice may transmit bubonic plague to other individuals). As the victim scratches the site of the wound, the bacilli multiply and spread to the lymph glands in the groin (in the case of a flea bite to the leg) or the armpits (in the case of a bite to the arm). As the immune system struggles to contain the infection, the lymph glands become swollen and inflamed, giving rise to the painful egg-shaped "buboes" from which the disease takes its name. On average, plague takes three to five days to incubate, and another three to five days before the victim dies (untreated, bubonic plague is fatal in around 60 percent of cases), the final stages being marked by extensive hemorrhaging and organ failure. In the most toxic form of bubonic plague, known as septicemic plague, the skin becomes mottled with dark blue patches and the extremities may turn black, hence one possible derivation of the disease's name, "Black Death." In the last stages of the infection, victims often fall into a delirium and are unable to bear the slightest touch to their sores. The only mercy is that this form of plague usually kills quickly and is only transmissible by bites from fleas.

By contrast, the pneumonic form can be spread directly from person to person and can arise either from inhalation of Y. *pestis* or septicemic spread of bacteria from the bubonic form of the disease. Typically, an originating case of pneumonic plague occurs when some of the bacilli escape the lymph system and migrate to the victim's lungs, causing edema and secondary infection (this is particularly common when a bubo forms in the neck region). During this time, the victim is noninfectious but may exhibit a fever and rapid pulse. Within one to four days, however, the victim's condition suddenly deteriorates as the edema spreads, triggering necrotizing pneumonia throughout the lungs and violent paroxysms. At this stage, the victim typically coughs or "spits" blood, causing the bed sheets to become spotted and stained crimson. Unless treated within twelve hours of the onset of fever, pneumonic plague is invariably fatal. Suspended in cough droplets or sputum, the bacilli can also be expelled as far as twelve inches, making it easy for someone lying on a nearby sofa or an adjacent bed to catch the disease. In cold weather and cool, humid conditions the bacilli can also become attached to water droplets and linger in the air for minutes or hours at a time. The bacteria can also survive for up to three days on hard surfaces, such as glass and steel, and for much longer in the soil and other organic material.

It is difficult to be certain what proportion of deaths that occurred during historical outbreaks were due to the bubonic as opposed to the pneumonic form of the disease, because prior to modern bacteriological tests diagnosis was uncertain and rested on the interpretation of clinical symptoms and signs. The first plague pandemic that began during the reign of the Byzantine emperor, Justinian I, and which is estimated to have killed some 25 million people throughout the Mediterranean basin between 541 and 750, is thought to have been largely bubonic. However, the second pandemic appears to have been a mixed outbreak. Colloquially known as the Black Death, the pandemic began in 1334 in China before spreading along the great trade routes to Constantinople, Florence, and other European capitals in the middle decades of the fourteenth century, reducing Europe's population by approximately one-quarter to one-half between 1347 and 1353 and killing at least 20 million people, possibly as many as 50 million. To judge by contemporary accounts, buboes and swellings, called *gavocciolo* by Italian chroniclers, were ubiquitous. However, in 1348, the first year of the Black Death in Europe, so were pneumonic symptoms. "Breath," wrote one Sicilian chronicler, "spread the infection among those speaking together . . . and it seemed as if the victim[s] were struck all at once by the affliction and [were] shattered by it. . . . Victims coughed up blood, and after three days of incessant vomiting for which there was no remedy, they died, and with them died not only everyone who talked with them, but also anyone who had acquired or touched or laid hands on their belongings."

The news that a deadly pathogen from the Middle Ages had arrived in the City of Angels was not something anyone in Los Angeles wanted to hear in 1924, least of all business leaders. As William Deverell, a historian of California and the West, puts it, at a time when Los Angeles was selling itself as a hygienic retirement destination, "plague was not the sort of thing expected in the proud city of tomorrow." Plague's presence in Los Angeles was also a considerable blow to the prestige of the US Public Health Service (PHS) and the Californian State Board of Health. Just ten years earlier, health officials had confidently declared that all "discoverable" plague had been eradicated from California. This announcement was based on the new knowledge of plague's ecology that had been acquired following the outbreaks of bubonic plague in San Francisco in the early years of the century.

Introduced to the city in around 1900, most likely from black rats that had hitched a ride to San Francisco on a steamship from Honolulu, the plague was at first confined to Chinatown, where it killed 113 people. However, following the earthquake and fire that struck San Francisco in 1906, rats were displaced from their downtown runs and dispersed throughout the city, sparking new outbreaks in 1907–1908 over a much wider urban area. In response, US Assistant Surgeon General Rupert Blue launched a massive rat extermination campaign. Whereas in 1903 Blue had concentrated on demolishing houses in Chinatown and baiting rat holes with arsenic, now he ordered his men to hunt down and kill rats wherever they found them. By January 1908, when the last two cases of bubonic plague were seen in the city, some two million rats had been exterminated and many thousands had been autopsied, giving Blue, and his chief laboratorian, George McCoy, new insights into the transmission of plague and its persistence in rodent reservoirs in interepidemic periods. Unlike in India and Asia, where the principal vector of plague was the black rat, *Rattus rattus*, Blue and McCoy discovered that in San Francisco the main vector had been the brown sewer rat, *Rattus norvegicus*. A prolific breeder, the brown rat's preferred habitat is sewers and cellars where it likes to lay out its run in the shape of a Y, with its food store hidden at one branch and its nest at the other—evidence, according to Blue, of the rodent's "sagacity" at evading predators. This strategy had served the brown rat well, enabling it to spread from the waterfront in northeast San Francisco as far as the County Hospital in the southwest.

Although in 1908 no one had definitively demonstrated that fleas living on rats were vectors of plague, their incriminating role was widely presumed, and Blue routinely ordered his men to comb rats for fleas and count the number of ectoparasites. He found that in winter his men could comb twenty rats and recover only one flea among them, but in warm weather the flea numbers multiplied, such that a healthy rat could harbor twenty-five fleas, while a sick one might host eighty-five. As long as these fleas fed on rats, they hypothesized, they posed little threat to human populations. It was only when rats were evicted from their runs and came into contact with people, or when plague-infected fleas killed their rodent hosts and began looking for a new blood meal, that humans risked being infected. However, there was much more to the ecology of plague than just rats and fleas.

In China, it had long been suspected that marmots acted as reservoirs of plague in interepidemic periods. However, until Blue, McCoy, and William Wherry, a bacteriologist with the San Francisco Board of Health, began studying sporadic outbreaks of plague in counties on the east side of San Francisco Bay in 1908, no one had suspected that Californian ground squirrels and other wild rodents indigenous to the western United States might be similarly susceptible to infection with *Y. pestis* or might play a similar role in maintaining transmission of the parasite in interepidemic periods. Blue's suspicions had first been aroused five years earlier when a blacksmith from Contra Costa County died of bubonic plague at a hospital in San Francisco. On questioning his friends and family, Blue learned that the blacksmith had not visited the city in over a month, but that three to four days before the onset of his illness he had shot and killed a ground squirrel in the hills near his home. By July 1908 Blue was certain that there were no more infected rats in San Francisco. However, that same month he learned that the son of a rancher from Concord in Contra Costa County had contracted plague and died, prompting Blue to dispatch his top rat catcher, William Colby Rucker, to investigate. The scene that greeted Colby at the ranch had all the hallmarks of a classic epizootic, with bodies of dead rats littering the ground. In a barn on the ranch near where the boy had died, Colby also recovered a dead squirrel. Blue immediately ordered Colby and his men to collect squirrels from other ranches in the region and discovered that several were infected with *Y. pestis*. As Blue later wrote Washington, DC, this was "perhaps the first demonstration of the occurrence in nature of bubonic plague in the ground squirrel (*Citellus beecheyi*) of California." McCoy speculated that the squirrels must have caught the plague from rats that had migrated from San Francisco to Oakland and had mingled with wild rodents in the hills behind Berkeley, exchanging ectoparasites in the process. Evidence for this hypothesis was supported by his discovery that the California ground squirrels were heavily infested with two species of flea, *Hoplopsyllus anomalus* and *Nosopsyllus fasciatus*. The latter was commonly found on rats and, together with *Xenopsylla cheopis*, the oriental rat flea, was thought to have been the principal vector of bubonic plague during the 1906 San Francisco outbreak. However, McCoy observed that the squirrel fleas also readily attacked humans, writing that at one point his "squirrel stock room became so heavily infested that upon going into the room one was certain to be bitten by many of the parasites." McCoy also found that in the laboratory it was easy to transmit plague by means of the *H. anomalus* flea from squirrels to guinea pigs and rats, and vice versa, leading him to conclude that "it is not improbable that the conveyance in nature is in the same way."

The discovery that squirrels might act as reservoirs of plague between rat epizootics and that their fleas might also be capable of transmitting the infection to humans caused Blue "considerable apprehension." However, it was thought that as long as the risk was confined to Contra Costa and Alameda Counties, there was little to worry about. Then in August, a report reached McCoy of the death of a ten-year-old boy in Elysian Park, in northeast Los Angeles, some four hundred miles to the south. On arriving at the boy's home, McCoy discovered that seven days before the onset of illness, the boy had come across a ground squirrel in his backyard and it had bitten him on the hand. Both the boy and a dead squirrel recovered from the property subsequently tested positive for plague. The boy's home, McCoy noted, was just two miles from city hall and backed onto the yards of the San Francisco–Los Angeles line of the Southern Pacific Railroad.*

This was alarming news and prompted the PHS to cast its net wider. After writing Washington for more rifles and ammunition, Blue sent hunting parties into nearby woodlands and hillsides to collect squirrels and bring them to McCoy's laboratory. By 1910, McCoy had examined 150,000 ground squirrels across ten California counties and discovered that 402, or 0.3 percent of them, were infected with plague. These diseased squirrels had been recovered from as far south as San Luis Obispo and the San Joaquin Valley, many miles from the sea and the presumed original ports of entry to the United States. In response, Blue focused his efforts on the areas where infected squirrels had been found, poisoning their burrows with carbon bisulfide and sending hunting parties into the woods to shoot stray rodents. Blue's war on rodents made him a household name, and in 1912 he was elevated to surgeon general, the top medical position in the country. In his absence, others carried on the eradication work he had begun, and by 1914 ground squirrels had been recovered from twenty-one infected ranches and their burrows so thoroughly poi-

---

* Though McCoy states that the squirrel had bitten the boy on the hand, he goes on to say that it is uncertain whether the boy contracted plague this way, speculating that he may have contracted it from infected fleas, which is the more usual transmission route of plague from squirrels to humans.

soned that officials were only able to find one infected squirrel when they repeated the survey, prompting Colby to claim that "danger of its further spread has been removed." But Colby and his colleagues were wrong. The ecology of plague was far more complex than they could have anticipated—as one expert put it, writing in 1949, plague was "like following the different voices in a Bach fugue," the difference being that while the structure of a Bach fugue is known, with plague "the basic design is unknown." The fact is, plague never entirely disappears from wild rodent populations. Rather, the pathogen circulates continually between fleas, squirrels, and other wild mammals, including chipmunks, marmots, and prairie dogs.* Many of these rodents have genetic or acquired immunity so are resistant to illness. However, every few years, this resistance wanes and the host population crashes, leaving fleas without a source of food. It is at this stage that the fleas seek a new host, seizing upon whatever animal happens to stray into the vacant rodents' burrows. This could be another species of ground squirrel or it could be a wild rat or a field mouse, or even a rabbit. Regardless, the transfer usually results in a violent epizootic as these new and highly susceptible hosts fall victim to the disease for the first time—hence the rats that Colby found littering the grounds of the ranch in Concord.

Nonetheless, there was good reason why, by 1924, California health officials should have been on their guard, not only against renewed outbreaks of the bubonic form of the disease, but of pneumonic plague, too. Indeed, bacteriologists only needed to recall the outbreak of pneumonic plague that had occurred in Oakland five years earlier, killing thirteen people. The outbreak began in August 1919 when an Italian man named Di Bortoli went hunting in the foothills of Ala-

---

* Rabbits, pigs, coyotes, bobcats, badgers, bears, gray foxes, and skunks can also be infected with plague, though they rarely exhibit symptoms. By contrast, domestic cats are highly susceptible.

meda County, returning with several squirrels for the table of his rooming house in Oakland. Within days, Di Bortoli was complaining of fever and pain in his right side and had reported to a doctor. Unfortunately, the physician attributed Bortoli's symptoms to influenza and even after Di Bortoli developed a painful bubo on his neck, the doctor did not think of plague. Most likely, it was septicemic spread of plague from this bubo that sparked a tonsillar infection and secondary pneumonia. The result was that by the time Di Bortoli died at the end of the month, five other people, including his landlady and a nurse, had been infected and by September 11, thirteen more people had contracted plague. In all, only one survived. Fortunately, thanks to the rapid hospitalization and isolation of the patients, the outbreak was self-limiting. Nevertheless, the fact that thirteen people had died and that the outbreak had begun following contact with a squirrel was extremely alarming, suggesting that, as with Siberian marmots, Californian squirrels might harbor fleas infected with highly virulent and potentially pneumotrophic strains of the bacillus. As William Kellogg, the director of the State Board of Health Bureau's communicable disease division, observed, "Until plague-infected ground squirrels are entirely eradicated from California we shall always have a sword of Damocles hanging over our heads."

Kellogg's concerns were born of bitter experience. In 1900 when plague had announced itself in San Francisco, it had been he who had taken samples from the lymph gland of the first presumed plague patient to Joseph Kinyoun at the United States' Marine Hospital laboratory on Angel Island for testing. After Kinyoun demonstrated that the tissues contained the plague bacillus, and that that organism caused guinea pigs to sicken and die, Kellogg then found himself thrust into the uncomfortable position of having to defend Kinyoun against a vitriolic campaign orchestrated by California's governor, Henry Gage, and local business interests. Angered by the imposition of the quarantine around Chinatown, Gage and his allies called into question Kinyoun's methods and findings, and alleged that the quarantine measures were a "scare." They also proposed that "it be made a felony to broadcast the presence of plague." Kinyoun's findings were subsequently upheld by a commission of prominent bacteriologists appointed by the US Treasury, but Kellogg, whose competence came in for similar scrutiny and who faced similar vilification, felt that "for unexampled bitterness, unfair and dishonest methods" the campaign "probably never had been and never again will be equaled."

Thankfully, the 1900 outbreak had been brought under control with just 121 cases and 113 deaths, and when plague revisited San Francisco in 1907 politicians and health officials no longer tried to pretend it was a fiction, moving swiftly to contain the disease by launching an extensive rat extermination campaign. Like other bacteriologists and officials who had been "blooded" by America's first experience of plague, Kellogg remained a keen student of the disease, and when in the winter of 1910 reports reached California of an outbreak of pneumonic plague in Manchuria, he followed news of the spreading outbreak keenly. Most likely sparked by tarbagans, a species of Mongolian and Siberian marmot valued for their fur, the epidemic appears to have begun at Manchouli, near the Chinese-Siberian border, in October 1910 before spreading via the trans-Manchurian railway to Harbin and other towns along the way. The principal culprits were inexperienced Chinese hunters who had been attracted to Manchuria by the high prices for pelts and did not take as much care as Manchurian trappers when handling sick tarbagans. As the Manchurian winter closed in and the hunters headed back to China, they mingled with returning agricultural workers and "coolies," crowding into packed railway carriages and inns. Soon, hospitals were overrun with patients, and by February 1911 some 50,000 people had died. Many of the bodies were cremated or dynamited in plague pits. According to Wu Lien-Teh, a Cambridge-educated Chinese plague expert who made a detailed study of the epidemic, reports of buboes were entirely absent, but pneumonic symptoms were ubiquitous. Working with the American physician and tropical medicine specialist Richard Strong, Wu performed twenty-five autopsies and used bacteriological techniques to confirm the presence of *Y. pestis*, subsequently presenting the evidence at the International Plague Conference called by the Chinese in Mukden in 1911.

At this time, most experts subscribed to the idea that plague was a rat-borne disease, most likely communicated by fleas, so the idea that the bacillus could be spread in droplet form directly to humans from tarbagans and marmots was controversial. But when the Chinese and Japanese authorities made a close examination of rats—some 50,000 were rounded up—they could not find any evidence of infection, and support for the theory grew. Some experts suspected the Manchurian strains were more virulent than those associated with previous bubonic outbreaks in India and elsewhere; others that the tarbagan-derived bacilli were pneumotrophic, meaning they had an affinity for the lungs. This theory received a boost when Strong, who headed the Biological Laboratory in Manila (part of the Philippine Bureau of Science) and led the American delegation to the conference, demonstrated that plague bacilli could be cultured from agar plates on which patients had been allowed to breathe, and that tarbagans could also be infected with pneumonic plague if exposed to the organism in droplet form.

Another compelling theory concerned the weather. In Manchuria the average temperature during the three months of the epidemic had been −30°C, whereas in India, where plague had raged on and off since 1896 and had been largely bubonic, the average temperature had been 30° C. Hypothesizing that the failure of pneumonic plague to spread in India had been due to the higher average temperatures there, Oscar Teague and M. A. Barber, two bacteriologists attached to the Philippine Bureau of Science, decided to perform a series of evaporation experiments with *Y. pestis* and other infectious bacteria. These showed that sprayed plague droplets disappeared very quickly from the atmosphere in conditions of low humidity, whereas the converse was the case in conditions of high humidity. "Such an atmosphere is, under ordinary circumstances, of common occurrence in very cold climates, whereas it is extremely rare in warm ones," they wrote. "Hence, since the droplets of sputum persist longer, the plague bacilli remain alive longer in the air, and there is a greater tendency for the disease to spread in cold climates than in warm ones."

Not everyone was persuaded by this argument, however, or convinced that climate had been the decisive factor. Though impressed by the cold weather in Harbin in 1910, Wu did not think it had played a major part in the Manchurian outbreak, pointing out that there was "ample evidence" to show that pneumonic outbreaks also occurred in regions with hot climates, such as Egypt and West Africa. Instead, Wu believed that the decisive factor had been the overcrowding and the proximity to infectious patients, pointing out that "most infections occurred indoors, specially at night-time, when the coolies returned to their warm but crowded shelters." Nor did he accept another theory according to which the cold weather had resulted in the wide dispersion of *frozen* particles of plague-infected sputum. "If infection occurred in the open, it certainly was a direct one from patient to patient, and did not result from inhalation of frozen particles of sputum," he stated.

Weighing the circumstances of the Oakland outbreak, Kellogg concluded that the health department had been fortunate that the outbreak had occurred in August, as the warm weather and low humidity meant that "conditions were not favorable for the transfer of infected droplets." The result was that "the drying and consequent death of the bacillus was so rapid that the ordinary measures of prophylaxis . . . sufficed to check the progress of the infection." Had the weather been cooler or the atmospheric water deficit lower, then things might have been different, he acknowledged, but that had not been and was unlikely to be the case in California. While San Francisco and Los

Angeles needed to be on their guard against further cases of bubonic plague sparked by stray squirrels, he concluded, it was cities in the East that should be most concerned about the pneumonic form of the disease. All it would take, he observed, was for someone to be infected by a squirrel and, while incubating the disease, journey to "some eastern state in winter time and [develop] an infection such as that of Di Bortoli." He concluded that while the persistence of sylvatic reservoirs of plague in California ground squirrels consituted a permanent risk of the bubonic form of the disease, the pneumonic form was "probably not a serious menace on the Pacific coast, owing to climatic conditions."

THE IDENTIFICATION OF *Y. pestis* in Horace Gutiérrez's sputum and the symptoms of severe pneumonia with bloody expectorations and cyanosis should have been a wake-up call that the improbable had happened and that pneumonic plague was at large in the Mexican quarter, even as Los Angeles broiled in a late fall heat wave. But that is not what happened. Instead, fearing the political and economic repercussions, not to mention the panic that might attend an official announcement that the Black Death had arrived in the city of the future, health officials prevaricated. On being shown the slide packed with rod-shaped bacteria, the city's health commissioner, Dr. Luther Powers, denied the evidence in front of his eyes, telling Maner the slide had been poorly prepared and that he needed to rerun the tests. Nevertheless, he took the precaution of sending quarantine officers to the Macy Street District, telling them there had been a "return of [Spanish] flu" in a virulent form in the Mexican quarter. By now, Maria Samarano, Guadalupe's 80-year-old grandmother—the woman whom Bogen had examined at Carmelita Street—had been admitted to County General, and on November 1 she died, becoming the fourth victim of the outbreak. But still no one dared utter the "p" word in public. However, the evening before, the hospital's superintendent had sent a telegram to state and federal officials asking where he might obtain plague serum and vaccine. One of the telegrams was intercepted by Benjamin Brown, the PHS's senior surgeon in Los Angeles. Not sure that he could trust what he was reading, Brown called the hospital to inquire if there were plague patients on its wards, then wired the Surgeon General, Hugh S. Cumming, to alert him to the gravity of the situation. Encoding his telegram for secrecy, he dictated: "Eighteen cases ekkil [pneumonic plague]. Three suspects. Ten begos [deaths]. Ethos [situation bad]. Recommend federal aid." In response, Cumming ordered James Perry, a senior surgeon stationed in San Francisco, to proceed to Los Angeles and make discreet inquiries, but by now quarantine officers were roping off the eight city blocks that encompassed the death house at Clara Street and newspapermen were asking questions.

Infectious diseases have long been objects of rumor and panic. When the identity of the pathogen is unknown or uncertain, and information about the outbreak is veiled in secrecy, these rumors—and the fears that attend them—can quickly spiral out of control. The first into print was the *Los Angeles Times*, posting a report on November 1 that nine mourners who had attended the wake at 742 Clara Street had died of a "strange malady" resembling pneumonia. Listing the victims by name, perhaps so its readers would have no doubt that, for the moment, this was a Hispanic rather than an Anglo-Saxon problem, the paper went on to report that eight more people were confined to the hospital's isolation ward and that some of these were also "expected to die." The paper also revealed that the health authorities had "isolated a germ" but, like the *Herald Examiner* and other Los Angeles papers, the *Times* avoided mentioning the dreaded word *plague*. Instead, the paper stated that there would be no official announcement until bacteriological studies had been concluded, and that for the moment patients had been given "the technical diagnosis of Spanish influenza." Incredibly, it was this or a similar coded report in another California paper that

seems to have alerted Kellogg's colleague, Dr. William Dickie, the secretary of the State Board of Health, that something was amiss in the
Mexican quarter. Dickie immediately sent a telegram to Dr. Elmer
Pascoe, Los Angeles's acting health officer, asking him to "Kindly wire
immediately cause of death of Lucena Samarano [sic]." Pascoe, who
had only just taken up the city's top health post following the sudden
death of the previous occupant from a heart attack, kept his answer
brief and to the point, "Death L.S. caused by *Bacillus pestis.*"

By now the quarantine had been extended to Belvedere Gardens,
confining some 4,000 people within the plague zone, and the police
and fire department had strict instructions not to let anyone in or out
of the roped-off area. In addition, guards had been posted at the front
and back of homes that were known to contain or that had formerly
contained plague victims. Public gatherings were also prohibited, and
parents were instructed to keep their children out of school and away
from movie houses. Even Pacific Electric trolley cars, which continued
to run along Macy Street, were banned from letting riders board or
alight at stops near the quarantined area.

This was Los Angeles's shark-in-the-water moment. The sight of
armed guards barring entry to the Mexican quarter was the equivalent of posting signs on the beach that it was no longer safe to enter
the sea. But rather than admitting the truth, city and health authorities, with the backing of local newspaper editors, sought to main-
tain the fiction that, as the *Los Angeles Times* put it, the outbreak was
merely a "malignant form of pneumonia." This infuriated *El Heraldo
de Mexico*, the Spanish language newspaper, which railed against "the
hermetic silence in which authorities have locked themselves." But
it was a lone voice and no other paper in Los Angeles dared mention plague. Outside Los Angeles, however, it was a different story.
"21 Victims of 'Black Death' in California," declared the Associated
Press on November 1. "Pneumonic Plague is Feared after 13 die in
Los Angeles," announced the *Washington Post* on November 2. "Pneu-

monic Plague takes seven more victims," reported the *New York Times* on November 3.

The contrasting treatment of the outbreak in America's metropolitan dailies perhaps says more about the rivalries between East and West Coast business elites, and commercial concerns about the plague's economic impacts, than it does about the competence of Los Angeles health officials. Faced with the publicity nightmare of a disease from the Dark Ages appearing in twentieth-century Los Angeles, it is little wonder that the first instinct of the city's civic leaders and their press allies was to obfuscate. As George Young, the managing editor of the *Herald Examiner*, informed the Board of Directors of the Los Angeles Chamber of Commerce, Hearst newspapers "would print nothing we didn't think was in the interests of the city." At stake was not merely the viability of Los Angeles's tourism industry and future real estate sales, but the ambition to make the Port of Los Angeles at San Pedro the largest commercial harbor in the United States. Should federal health officials in Washington suspect plague was anywhere near the port, the surgeon general would have no choice but to close the harbor and impose a strict maritime quarantine. Once a quarantine had been instituted it would continue for at least ten days and could only be lifted when the authorities were sure the city was free of plague and there was no danger of the disease being reintroduced to wharfside areas by rats and other rodents. But by that point, of course, the damage to the city's reputation would have been done.

By contrast, for the New York newspapers there was nothing like plague to boost circulation, especially when the outbreak lay a safe 3,000 miles to the west. Besides, for years Los Angeles had boasted of its superior climate and quality of life, bombarding easterners with postcards adorned with sun-kissed orange groves and preternaturally happy couples. Never mind if reporting the truth fostered panic: it was worth it just to puncture the booster hubris and wipe the smirk off those sunny Californian faces.

⊰≫⊱

IN 1924 there was no treatment or cure for pneumonic plague. The best that physicians could offer were stimulants such as caffeine and digitalis, or depressants, such as morphine. In theory, vaccines containing killed bacteria or convalescent serums containing antibodies from patients who had survived infection with plague might have made a difference, but only if convalescents with immunity to the disease could be found in time and the serums administered early enough in the infection to make a difference to the course of the disease. In the absence of such measures, 90 percent of infections were fatal.

For those who had attended Luciana Samarano's wake, had boarded in her rooming house, or who had helped care for one of her sick or dying relatives, it was almost certainly too late. But for those who had not yet been exposed to infectious sputum or blood from the Samaranos' extended family, there was one measure that was certain to break the chain of infections: quarantine and the rapid isolation of the sick. These measures had eventually halted the outbreak in Harbin in 1911, and they had also stemmed the outbreak in Oakland in 1919. Even without an official diagnosis of plague, physicians at County General were sufficiently wary of the infection and the alarming symptoms of cyanosis to place patients in an isolation ward and wear masks and rubber gloves when approaching their beds. However, the decision to quarantine Macy Street and Belvedere Gardens appears to have had little to do with infection control and everything to do with racism and prejudice.

Reconstructing the precise sequence of events is difficult given the incomplete documentation and the lack of transparency by the Los Angeles newspapers and Mayor George Cryer. But what is certain is that only Walter Dickie, the secretary of the State Board of Health, had the legal authority to order a quarantine of the Mexican quarter and he did not learn about the outbreak until November 1, by which time, of course, the area had already been roped off. Instead, it seems that the decision was made by the county health chief, J. L. Pomeroy, acting on his own initiative. Though Pomeroy was a qualified doctor, his decision appears to have had less to do with his knowledge of plague than his experience of previous quarantines and his low regard for Mexicans. By the 1920s ethnic quarantines, spurred by fears of small-pox and typhus being introduced by migrants from across the border, had become a routine measure in Los Angeles and other southern Californian towns. According to Pomeroy, special guard details were "the only effective way of quarantining Mexicans," and he ordered his men to institute the quarantine by stealth so as not to spread alarm. To this end, Pomeroy conscripted seventy-five police officers and positioned his men discreetly at the boundaries of Macy Street and Carmelita Street in Belvedere Gardens. To avoid "a general stampede," he instructed the guards to wait until after midnight when they were certain all residents had returned home. It was only then that ropes were strung around the zone and the "quarantine was [made] absolute." The measures, which were in force for two weeks, would eventually extend to five urban districts in which Hispanics were known to reside. However, only two of these, Macy Street and Belvedere, had verifiable cases of plague. As Deverell puts it, "the others had only verified cases of ethnicity. In other words, Mexicans lived there."

Though judged by today's standards Pomeroy's methods were discriminatory, they appear to have been extremely effective. With the exception of an ambulance driver who ferried one of the patients to the hospital, all the casualties, bar one, came from within the quarantine zone and could be traced to the Samarano clan or to mourners who had been present at one of the wakes. Indeed, Pomeroy's decision to impose a quarantine seems to have been prompted in part by the questioning of boarders who shared the house at 343 Carmelita Street with Guadalupe's elderly mother, Maria Samarano. This was the address that Bogen had visited two days earlier and where he had discovered Maria and Guadalupe's brother, Victor, lying deathly ill. By the time Pomeroy arrived at Carmelita Street, Victor was dead of suspected "meningitis." However, on quizzing the other boarders and learning that Victor had recently attended his father's funeral, Pomeroy immediately posted armed guards at the front and back of the house. Next, he discovered that one of Luciana Samarano's cousins had died at another house in Belvedere Gardens and that his wife was also ill with what was presumed to be the same disease. This was the flag that appears to have convinced Pomeroy to draw a wider line around Macy District and extend the quarantine to Belvedere Gardens, even though it lay across the city line in Los Angeles County.

Waking the following morning to find that they were effectively prisoners—"inmates" was the official term used by the health authorities—must have been a terrifying experience for the Mexican residents and anyone else caught up in the dragnet. Indeed, no sooner was the quarantine in place than the authorities began house-to-house inspections. Those who were sick or were suspected of having been in contact with sick persons were removed to the isolation ward at County General, while those left behind were told to prepare a mixture of hot water, salt, and lime juice, and gargle with it several times a day. The chamber of commerce refused to requisition additional funds to provide provisions for the trapped residents of the plague zone. Instead, it was left to local charities to deliver packages of food and milk to stricken families.

Confined to their homes, waiting to see who would be next to succumb to the *Muerto Negro*, as Spanish speakers referred to the disease, one can only imagine the images that flashed through people's minds and the thoughts that they clung to for comfort. As Camus reminds us, in such situations "we tell ourselves that pestilence is a mere bogy of the mind, a bad dream that will pass away." But the plague was not a bogy, it was real and it could strike, without warning, at any time. The only mercy was that the worst suffering took place far from the quarantine zone inside the isolation ward at County General. There, in a desperate effort to halt the course of the disease, doctors placed patients on an intravenous drip of Mercurochrome solution, a mercury-based antiseptic used to treat minor cuts and bruises that was almost certainly useless against plague.* The first to receive the treatment was ten-year-old Roberto Samarano, the eldest of Guadalupe's three sons. He was hooked up to a Mercurochrome drip on October 28 and given three successive injections, only to die two days later, his body "practically riddled with plague infection." Roberto's death was followed by that of his younger brother, Gilberto, and Alfredo Burnett, Luciana Samarano's son from an earlier marriage (Alfredo died on November 11 after a heroic thirteen-day struggle with the disease that saw him slipping in and out of a "restless delirium"). By now two boarders at 742 Clara Street had also died. Incredibly, the only member of the Samarano clan to survive the death house was the Samaranos' second son, Raul. The eight-year-old was evacuated from Clara Street at the same time as his siblings, but, unlike his brothers, was given plague serum. He lived, growing up to enjoy a career in the navy and the Los Angeles Army Corps of Engineers. Another notable survivor was Mary Costello, a nurse who had attended Guadalupe Samarano at Clara Street. Costello was admitted to County General on October 29. By Halloween both her lungs were showing signs of consolidation and she was bringing up "bloody expectorations," but after being given Mercurochrome solution Costello showed a slight improvement, and a few days later she also received plague serum. It was this that may have made the difference.

Incredible as it might seem today, Angelenos in other parts of the city appear to have been largely ignorant of the outbreak and the sig-

---

* Mercurochrome is the brand name for dibromohydroxymercurifluorescein, sometimes called merbromin. Its use was discontinued by the FDA in 1998 because of fears of potential mercury poisoning.

nificance of the quarantine. One man recalled the plague as "a big hush-up," while his father, who lived within walking distance of Macy Street and was a regular reader of the *Los Angeles Times*, admitted he had known little about the outbreak. This is not surprising when you consider that the *Los Angeles Times* and other municipal papers did not refer to the disease by its proper name until November 6, by which time the epidemic had more or less run its course. Even then, they sought to justify their evasion by adding that pneumonic plague was merely the "technical term" for malignant pneumonia. Plague was "not a new phenomenon in California," Dickie pointed out truthfully, if a little disingenuously. "While an outbreak of plague is always a potential menace . . . there is no reason for public alarm."

Outside of Los Angeles, however, it was a different story, as newspapers competed to keep their readers abreast of the latest developments. The call for plague serum and the news of its dramatic journey received particular attention, not least of all because the manufacturer, Mulford Laboratories of Philadelphia, used Los Angeles's plight as a marketing opportunity to issue regular press updates on the progress of the serum from the West to the East Coast. Pascoe's appeal for serum had reached Mulford on November 3, prompting the company to dispatch several vials by automobile to Mineola airfield in Long Island. The following day the serum was transferred to a mail plane and flown 3,000 miles to San Francisco and thence to Los Angeles, reaching the city health department on November 5. "Serum for plague speeds by plane to Los Angeles" reported the New York *Evening World News* on November 5; "5000 more doses of serum go west," added the *Public Ledger* of Philadelphia a few days later. Mulford did its best to play up the "thrilling" story of the vaccine's bicoastal journey, describing how within thirty-six hours of receiving the appeal, "the vials of serum were brought to the front lines where the battle is on against the Terror." Speed laws were "forgotten" as the precious vials were rushed to Mineola and, though the mail plane was briefly delayed by a storm at Salt Lake City, it was not long before "the messenger of mercy had right of way" again. Reading Mulford's sensational, self-serving prose must have been an uncomfortable experience for Los Angeles's own boosters. "It was pneumonic plague or Black Plague—the scourge of the fourteenth century," declared an announcement in the Mulford company journal, "the dread disease which numbered its victims by the millions." But Los Angeles business leaders were nothing if not adept at inoculating negative publicity, and soon they were putting their own spin on the episode, reassuring easterners that, as William Lacy, the president of the Los Angeles Chamber of Commerce, put it in an article in the *Los Angeles Realtor*, the city had suffered "a slight epidemic of pneumonic plague" and there was no reason for anyone to cancel their vacation plans.

If the outbreak challenged Los Angeles's carefully cultivated image as an idyllic holiday destination, it was no less of a headache for the State Board of Health and the PHS. In Washington the sensational newspaper reports were read with mounting alarm, leading to demands for reassurance from Congress that federal health officials were doing their utmost to ensure that plague did not spread to other harbor cities. The problem was that, technically, the outbreak in the Mexican quarter was the responsibility of the Los Angeles City Health department and the State Board of Health. Unless and until the outbreak reached the Port of Los Angeles, the PHS had no authority to intervene and could only serve in an advisory capacity. In theory, cooperation was in the interests of bureaucrats at the local, state, and federal level, but the city health commissioner was a political appointee who reported directly to the mayor, George Cryer, who in turn answered to the board of the chamber of commerce. This placed Pascoe in an impossible position, since Cryer was acutely sensitive to any statement that adversely impacted the city's image and its commercial prospects. Indeed, when Pascoe overstepped his authority by confirming to the eastern papers that the outbreak was due to pneumonic plague, Cryer passed him over for promotion and appointed a more pliant official to head the department. However, Dickie valued Pascoe's expertise and when, on November 3, at a meeting in Cryer's office, Dickie was put in charge of the plague cleanup operation, he insisted that Pascoe join his team. It would seem that Cryer had little choice but to accede to this demand; nor could he prevent Dickie offering a place on the advisory committee to James Perry, the PHS surgeon who had been dispatched from San Francisco to monitor the situation, despite the board's paranoia about word reaching Washington that plague might be encroaching on the environs of the port at San Pedro. Perry found himself in a similarly awkward position vis-à-vis his superiors in Washington, as he had to balance the surgeon general's concerns that local officials were not up to the job, against interventions that might be seen as interfering with the state's jurisdiction and undermining Dickie's authority. Indeed, it would seem that Perry may have gone too far in accommodating local officials, because on November 7, after being reprimanded for not transmitting information to Washington quickly enough, he explained that Dickie was "keenly desirous" of taking full control himself and that, in any case, there had been some doubt as to whether the outbreak was due to pneumonic plague. Interestingly, it would appear that Perry's skepticism was also the opinion of other experts, including Kellogg, who had accompanied him to Los Angeles and who had insisted on preparing fresh bacteriological slides before accepting Maner's diagnosis. Once it became clear that the outbreak was plague and deserved to be treated as such, however, Perry found himself increasingly at odds with Dickie. At the heart of their differences was the question whether the outbreak in the Mexican quarter was due to squirrels or rats, or some combination of both, and the implication that this might have for other parts of the city, including the port. Dickie and his colleagues in the county health department believed the epidemic would eventually be traced to infected squirrels, as had been the case with the Oakland outbreak, meaning that it should end when the last infectious patient had been isolated in the hospital. Indeed, when, at the suggestion of Karl Meyer, a bacteriologist who directed the Hooper Foundation for Medical Research in San Francisco and who had visited McCoy's plague laboratory to familiarize himself with his techniques, they combed rats in the Mexican quarter for fleas, they discovered a fair number harbored *H. anomalus* plus another species, *Diamanus montanus*, more commonly found on ground squirrels. Recalling the case of the boy in Elysian Park who had died of plague after exposure to a squirrel in 1908, Meyer suggested that this meant the outbreak had probably originated in the "hinterland," not the port. Perry thought otherwise and, responding to increasingly stern telegrams from Washington, insisted that the outbreak had been due to rats and that only a well-financed rodent eradication campaign targeting both the Mexican quarter and the port would be certain to rid Los Angeles of the disease. This was not a verdict the chamber of commerce wished to hear for obvious reasons. Nevertheless, in mid-November the chamber granted $250,000 to finance rodent extermination measures, with the promise of more money should it be needed. The pivotal decision came at a meeting of the chamber and the city council on November 13 when, standing in front of a map of greater Los Angeles studded with black pins representing pneumonic plague cases, Dickie warned: "I realize that the dream of Los Angeles and the dream of officials and the chamber of commerce is the harbor. Your dream will never come true as long as plague exists in Los Angeles and as long as there is any question of doubt in reference to the harbor." Unless San Pedro received a clean bill of health "half of the commerce of your harbor will quickly vanish," Dickie predicted, before concluding that "no disease known has such an effect upon the business world as the plague."

Los Angeles business leaders must have hoped that by granting substantial monies for antiplague measures, they would convince officials in Washington they were serious about addressing the rat problem and avoid the need for San Pedro to be quarantined. If so, their hopes were dashed. This had little to do with the enthusiasm with which Dickie and the City Health Department prosecuted rodent extermination, and everything to do with the PHS's concern for its reputation and its suspicion of California politicians and local business leaders. During the rat cleanup campaign in San Francisco, federal health officials had watched aghast as local newspapers, encouraged by Gage, had questioned Kinyoun's scientific competence. In the end, the reappearance of plague in San Francisco in 1907 had forced Gage to bow to the authority of the federal plague commission and cooperate with the PHS, but the experience had left Blue and Hugh Cumming, his successor as surgeon general who had been a protégé of Kinyoun's, suspicious of local city health departments and state-appointed health officials. In an attempt to foster closer cooperation between state and federal officials and improve the flow of information to Washington, in 1923 Cumming divided the country into seven public health districts and appointed experienced officers to each. One of the key postings was at the quarantine station at Angel Island, a position which went to Cumming's close friend and confidant, Assistant Surgeon General Richard H. Creel. From San Francisco, Creel would oversee quarantines for all ports along the United States' western seaboard, including Los Angeles, and keep a close eye on the progress of Dickie's campaign, feeding the information back to Cumming in Washington.

Determined to show that the State Board of Health was up to the task, Dickie moved into the new Pacific Finance Building off Wilshire Boulevard, where he fashioned himself "commander-in-chief." There, surrounded by color-coded maps studded with pins recording the locations of trapped rodents (red for rats, yellow for squirrels), he presided over 127 rodent exterminators. Under Dickie's direction, the campaign took on the trappings of a military exercise. One team of rat catchers was assigned exclusively to the harbor, with orders to inspect every arriving vessel and tag any rodent found in the vicinity of the port. The rats would then be removed to the city laboratory on Eighth Street for testing. At the same time, other squads fanned out across the Mexican quarter, performing "plague abatements." Modeled on the campaign in San Francisco's Chinatown in 1900, these involved removing the sidings from houses in and around Clara Street and raising the dwellings eighteen inches off the ground, so that dogs and cats could freely enter the buildings and flush diseased rodents from their lairs. At the same time, premises were ruthlessly stripped of furniture, clothing, and bedding, and funeral pyres made of tenants' belongings. These slash-and-burn tactics culminated with fumigation with petroleum, sulfur, or cyanide gas, measures that guaranteed that no creature foolish enough to return to the properties would survive long in the poisoned rooms. Running alongside these plague abatement measures was an equally ferocious rodent trapping and extermination campaign. Squares of bread baited with phosphorus or arsenic were scattered in suspect neighborhoods both inside and outside the quarantine zone. The city health department also offered a bounty of $1 for every dead rat or squirrel brought for counting and testing to its laboratory at Eighth Street. When this did not yield a sufficient bounty of rodents, the health department offered men a fixed salary of $130 a day. For First World War veterans this was considerably more than they could hope to earn in civilian employment, and soon the hunting parties were swelled by former infantrymen eager to demonstrate their sharpshooting skills. It was not long before Macy District echoed to the continuous pop of rifles, and when the hunting parties ran out of rodents within the city limits they fanned out to Belvedere Gardens and other areas in the county. "These surveys may take us a hundred miles or more from Los Angeles before we find the guilty rodent," Dickie warned.

Ironically, this campaign turned up far fewer rats in the Mexican quarter than had been expected, and virtually none in the harbor area. Indeed, by November 22, not one of the 1,000 rats trapped in the harbor had tested positive for plague. By contrast, to the embarrassment of the chamber of commerce, rats were readily trapped in the downtown blocks that housed the city's premier hotels and department stores. Meyer, who accompanied health officials on several of their inspections, recalled how at one downtown rice-cake factory run by a Japanese gentleman he had only to drop a crumb on the floor to "see a rat come up and pick it up." To Meyer, the scene was like something out of "Zanzibar" with the smart facades concealing a "jungle." The only way to ensure that such premises were rat-proof, he observed, was to pour concrete over the dirt floors, but that was expensive (and not always effective either).

By the end of the year, Dickie could boast that his men had trapped more than 25,000 rats and 768 squirrels. In addition, flooring and planking had been removed from countless buildings in and around Clara and Macy Streets, and poison laid at 1,000 premises. However, for all the intensity of the plague abatement measures, Perry was unimpressed by Dickie's efforts, informing Cumming that the Board's campaign had been "casual and periodic" and that its laboratory work could not be trusted. "It is apparent that Dr. Dickie does not appreciate the gravity of the situation, or the importance of enlarging the scope of the campaign, or of increasing the efficiency of the operations," Perry informed Cumming in mid-December. "This is evidenced by his non-acceptance of the proffered, concrete Service aid." Instead, he urged Cumming to dissociate the PHS from the state's program, warning that unless the PHS took charge of the campaign there was a "grave" danger the disease could spread to other countries. This was the one thing that Cumming could not allow, as under the provisions of the 1922 International Sanitary Convention the United States had a duty to ensure that "adequate measures" were being taken to prevent the spread of plague to other jurisdictions, failure to do so running the risk that foreign governments would impose quarantines against American shipping. Adding to Cumming's concern was the discovery of plague-infected rats in both New Orleans and Oakland. In the case of New Orleans, it was suspected the culprit had been the *Atlanticos*, a coal-steamer that had reached the Crescent City at the end of October after sailing from Oran, a notorious Algerian plague port that would be immortalized in Camus's 1947 novel. On board was a stowaway with a swelling on his groin. The stowaway was hospitalized and the ship fumigated, but soon after, eight plague rats were found on the waterfront, prompting the Louisiana State Board of Health to request the PHS begin a rodent survey. In the case of Oakland, there was no evidence of foreign introduction of plague. Instead, the alarm was raised by the discovery on December 13 of a plague rat on a garbage dump close to the waterfront.

In Los Angeles, by contrast, no plague-carrying rats had been found in the immediate vicinity of the harbor. However, by the end of December thirty-five had been retrieved from ranches within a mile of the port, and nearly twice as many again from other areas within a forty-mile circumference of San Pedro. In addition, survey squads had established that 64 percent of rats in the Los Angeles area were colonized by squirrel fleas and, although hunting parties had failed to turn up any infected squirrels in or around the city, eight squirrels retrieved from a ranch in San Luis Obispo that had been the focus of previous plague epizootics also tested positive for *Y. pestis*. At the same time, ranchers reported having observed epizootics of squirrel plague in San Benito and Monterey Counties the previous summer, suggesting that, as Meyer put it, 1924 had "truly [been] a sylvatic plague year in California." However, it was the reports from Europe of a new outbreak of rat plague at several Mediterranean ports that persuaded Cumming the PHS was facing a worldwide recrudescence of the disease and prompted him to finally institute quarantines at San Pedro and other "plague-infected" American ports.

Cumming's decision prompted a subtle but significant shift in the medical language. It was no longer the threat of domestic American squirrels transmitting the pneumonic form of the disease that was to be feared, so much as foreign introductions by "bubonic rats." That hysterical conjunction was sufficient to panic Congress into voting an emergency appropriation of $275,000 to support the PHS's renewed campaign against its old enemy. At first, Los Angeles's chamber of commerce protested the decision, accusing Cumming of "discriminatory" action since no plague rats had been found at San Pedro. In any case, it argued, while the harbor was the Fed's fiefdom, the port was the jurisdiction of the state and the city health department. For a while Cryer tried to argue the case for his new appointee, city health officer George Parrish. However, when Cryer got his wish and the city council authorized Parrish to take over the eradication campaign from Dickie, it also slashed his budget, forcing Cryer to swallow his pride and go cap in hand to President Calvin Coolidge to request that the PHS be allowed to assume responsibility for the plague cleanup work. As far as Cumming was concerned, there was only one man for the job, his predecessor Rupert Blue, who was promptly recommissioned into the Service and dispatched to Los Angeles. For Blue it was an opportunity to finish the work he had begun in 1908, and by July he was once again in his element, probing Los Angeles's downtown rat runs, overseeing the concreting over of basements and taking other abatement measures. "Nine suspicious rats and five ground squirrels have been found since June thirteen in widely separated sections, extending from Hollywood north to West Washington Street south," he wired Cumming on June 26. "Should these prove positive for plague we may expect several human cases to occur at any time. Seasonal conditions highly favorable for a return of the epidemic."

It is hard to say who deserves most credit for the eventual eradication of plague in Los Angeles, Blue or Dickie. The last reported case of pneumonic plague occurred on January 12, 1925, and, despite Blue's ominous telegram, the last plague-infected rat was recovered from eastern Los Angeles on May 21, in other words two months before

Blue took charge. And while Dickie may have been guilty of colluding in the press cover-up, he never doubted that the outbreak was serious. Moreover, his prompt action in quarantining Macy District and directing the plague cleanup efforts, however harsh and unfair the measures must have seemed to the area's Mexican residents, ensured that pneumonic plague did not spread to other parts of the city. Indeed, it could be argued that the Board's response might have been even more effective had the city health department alerted Dickie to the outbreak sooner, rather than waiting for him to learn about it from a newspaper. As Dickie observed in his official report on the outbreak, physicians and bacteriologists at County General were also culpable in failing to recognize the symptoms of plague in Jesus Lajun.* Though official figures probably did not reflect the full extent of the outbreak, in total there had been just forty-one cases of pneumonic plague and thirty-seven fatalities. In addition, there had been seven cases and five deaths from bubonic plague and a single fatal case of septicemic plague. Most important of all, perhaps, it was the last recorded outbreak of pneumonic plague anywhere in North America.

THE LOS ANGELES OUTBREAK upset the assumptions of Kellogg and other plague experts, challenging the wisdom that California's mild, year-round Mediterranean climate was a protection. Instead, it demonstrated that conditions of low humidity and warm weather made little difference to the transmission of the pneumonic form of the disease and that in Southern California the pathogen could assume as deadly a form as plagues during earlier historical periods. Indeed, the crucial factor was not the weather but the close proximity of the sick to

---

* The swelling in Jesus's groin was almost certainly an inguinal bubo that had been allowed to drain for three weeks before anyone thought to examine it for plague bacilli. A culture subsequently revealed "bipoloar organisms," and when a laboratory animal was inoculated with the culture it died within twelve hours.

the healthy. In the overcrowded conditions of the Mexican quarter the bacillus had found the ideal conditions for spread via respiratory drop-lets. Plague's explosive potential had been further amplified by burial rituals—in particular, the Catholic custom of holding open wakes—which brought mourners into close contact with infectious cadavers and those who might be incubating the infection. The Los Angeles outbreak had another legacy too: it shattered the belief that plague was largely a rat-borne disease of urban areas and that to eradicate it all you needed to do was clean up the places where rats bred. Though it was never proven that squirrels were the source of the 1924 outbreak, the discovery of squirrel fleas on rats recovered from the greater Los Ange-les area, together with the fact that no plague-infected rat was found between the port and the Mexican quarter, suggested that Meyer had been right and that the disease had most likely found its way to the Mexican quarter from the hinterland. Looking back, the signs had been there in 1908 when the boy in Elysian Park, thirty miles from the port, had died of plague after handling an infected squirrel in his backyard. It was around this time that squirrel die-offs had been reported in San Luis Obispo, a phenomenon that was repeated in 1924 when similar epizootics were observed in several counties in south-ern and northern California. Perhaps squirrels had originally caught the bug from rats rummaging in garbage dumps in Oakland, or that had hitched a ride south on the Southern Pacific Railroad. Or per-haps ground squirrels and other wild rodents had been harboring the plague bacillus for decades without anyone noticing. Whatever had been the case, the Los Angeles outbreak prompted Meyer and oth-ers to take a closer look at the role of squirrels in the persistence of plague between epidemics and the role of their fleas in the transmis-sion of the disease to rats and other wild rodents. With Dickie's help Meyer examined the records of previous outbreaks, trying to see if there was a relationship between epizootics observed in squirrels and human outbreaks. In 1927, when the state resumed responsibility for plague control work, Meyer and Dickie joined forces to survey ranches and woodlands suspected of harboring plague-infected squirrels. By the mid-1930s, state survey crews had trapped tens of thousands of squirrels and combed their fur for fleas, returning the rodents and their ectoparasites to Meyer's laboratory at the Hooper Foundation. Although many of these squirrels appeared perfectly healthy, Meyer discovered that some harbored latent infections and that their ground-up organs could be used to communicate plague to guinea pigs. Many were also infested with plague fleas. In addition, crews recovered diseased fleas from burrows that were known to have harbored infected squirrels twenty years previously but which were now occupied by other rodents, suggesting that in certain parts of the state ground squirrels constituted a hidden "reservoir" of disease. It was the beginning of a new ecological approach, one that by the mid-1930s would see Meyer adopt the term *sylvatic plague* to describe the preservation of the disease by forest-dwelling rodents.

By 1935, the PHS had joined the survey effort and established that sylvatic plague was endemic to eleven Pacific coast and Rocky Mountain states and that its reservoirs included eighteen species of ground squirrel, plus chipmunks, prairie dogs, marmots, wild rats, white-footed mice, kangaroo rats, and cottontails. By 1938 more than 100,000 squirrels had been trapped and shipped to the Hooper Foundation for examination. However, when Meyer came to autopsy the rodents he found that only a small percentage were infected with *Y. pestis*. He also observed that no sooner had the squirrels been eliminated than field mice took up residence in the empty burrows where they promptly became infested with the same plague fleas and "peddled" the infection to other rodents. Eradication was doomed to failure because sylvatic plague was "independent of the usual lines of communication," he concluded. The challenge was to keep sylvatic plague at a low level by periodically culling the squirrel populations that harbored *Y. pestis*. Of course, every now and again, someone might be bitten by a squirrel flea and contract the disease, but such events were rare, and as long as squirrels were prevented from infecting urban rat populations, sylvatic plague posed little threat to people living in built-up areas.

This is pretty much the approach employed by the CDC today. From its wildlife station in Fort Collins, Colorado, the CDC monitors the incidence of plague in prairie dogs, thought to be a key reservoir of plague in the western United States, and the spillover of the disease into squirrels and other wild rodents. In the Pacific Coast and Rocky Mountain states the principal vector is a species of flea called *Oropsylla montana*. Unlike in the rat flea *X. cheopis*, the midgut of *O. montana* gets blocked only rarely when it takes a blood meal, but it is known to unleash rapidly moving epizoonotics among Californian ground squirrels and rock squirrels through an "early-phase" transmission system.* When plague levels are considered dangerously high, warnings are posted in state parks and campgrounds showing a squirrel in a red circle with a diagonal slash through it. At such times hikers are warned not to feed squirrels and pet owners are advised to keep an eye on cats and other domestic animals lest they cross paths with a squirrel and accidentally become infested with their fleas. In spite of these precautions, every year about three people in the United States are infected with plague and in some years, as in 2006, there have been as many as seventeen infections. Prompt treatment with a powerful antibiotic, such as doxycycline or ciprofloxacin, is usually sufficient to clear the plague bacillus from the system.† Nonetheless, newspapers continue to run panicked headlines about the deaths of Americans from "bubonic plague" and the threats posed by squirrels and other

---

* Plague bacilli multiply rapidly in *X. cheopis*, sometimes causing blockages that prevent ingested blood from reaching the flea's midgut. These blockages cause the flea to feed more voraciously, thereby increasing the chances it will retransmit the infection.

† In patients treated with antibiotics the average fatality rate is 16 percent. In the untreated, it ranges from 66 to 93 percent.

wild rodents, as occurred in 2015 when an elderly Utah man died from the disease.

No one is sure what causes these periodic flare-ups, but climate and topography are thought to be important factors. Plague persists in relatively small geographical pockets, such as the high plateaus and grasslands of New Mexico, Utah, and Colorado, and the coastal fog belts of northern California, where the weather tends to be cool and damp year round. Indeed, in California, only the dry, central desert region is completely free of sylvatic plague. By contrast, in Yosemite National Park and other wilderness and coastal areas, plague is nearly always present. In such locales, it finds the ideal ecological balance between climate, flea vectors, and rodent hosts. It is only when unusual rainfall levels boost plant growth or some other factor increases the rodent and flea populations, that the balance between parasite and host is disturbed and plague risks spilling over into other animals.

Indeed, with the ongoing encroachment of residential developments into these wild habitats, the animal that most threatens to disturb this balance today is humans, which is why in the future we should expect further small outbreaks of plague, in its bubonic form at least. However, it is highly unlikely that Los Angeles or any other American city will ever again be confronted with an epidemic of pneumonic plague, much less a pandemic on the scale of the Black Death.

CHAPTER III

THE GREAT PARROT FEVER PANDEMIC

"What men against death have done."

—PAUL DE KRUIF

O n January 6, 1930, Dr. Willis P. Martin paid an urgent house call on a family in Annapolis, Maryland. Lillian, her daughter Edith, and Edith's husband Lee Kalmey, the owner of a local auto repair shop, had begun to feel feverish shortly after Christmas, and all three were now deathly ill. At first, they attributed their symptoms to influenza and the depressive effects of the recent stock market crash, which had hit Kalmey's business as hard as any, but in the first week of the new year their condition had taken a decided turn for the worse. To the chills and generalized aches and pains typical of influenza was now added an irritable dry cough, accompanied by constipation and exhaustion that alternated with headaches and insomnia. For large parts of the day, Lillian, Edith, and Lee lay somnolent as logs, the silence broken only by their intermittent mutterings. By contrast, when awake they would be restless and prone to fits of violent excitement. The most worrying symptom of all, however, was the rattling sound coming from deep within their lungs.

Dr. Martin suspected pneumonia, possibly mixed with typhoid fever. However, Lillian's husband, who had eaten the same meals as the rest of the family, was perfectly well, which tended to rule out a food-borne illness. The only other member of the household who had been sick was a parrot that Lillian's husband had purchased from a pet store in Baltimore and which Edith and Lee had kept at their home in the run-up to the Yuletide festivities so as to present the bird to Lillian as a surprise on Christmas Day. Unfortunately, by Christmas Eve the parrot's plumage had grown ruffled and dirty and the creature was showing signs of listlessness. Come Christmas Day the parrot was dead.

Dr. Martin was baffled by the family's symptoms and shared his bewilderment with his wife. At first, Mrs. Martin was similarly puzzled. Then Dr. Martin mentioned the dead parrot. It might be a coincidence, she said, but the previous Sunday she had been reading about an outbreak of "parrot fever" in a theatrical troupe in Buenos Aires. According to the newspaper report, the disease was being blamed for the death of two members of the company, who, in common with other members of the cast, had been required to interact with a live parrot on stage. That bird was now dead and pet owners throughout Argentina were being warned to report sickly psittacines—birds in the parrot family—to the authorities.

It sounded unlikely, ridiculous even, but Martin was not the type to take a chance. Instead, he sent a telegram to the PHS in Washington, DC:

REQUEST INFORMATION REGARDING DIAGNOSIS PARROT FEVER . . . WHAT INFORMATION AVAILABLE REGARDING PREVENTION SPREAD OF PARROT FEVER. . . . CAN YOU PLACE SUPPLY PARROT FEVER SERUM OUR DISPOSAL IMMEDIATELY. WIRE REPLY.

Martin was not the only doctor puzzled by the sudden appearance of mysterious pneumonias accompanied by typhoid-like symptoms in the United States that winter. By now similar telegrams were arriving at the PHS from Baltimore and New York, and health officials in

Ohio and California were fielding similar requests for information. Like Martin's telegram, these communications ended up on the desk of Surgeon General Hugh S. Cumming, who passed them on to his subordinate, Dr. George W. McCoy, the director of PHS's Hygienic Laboratory. A veteran of the bubonic plague investigations in San Francisco, McCoy was renowned for discovering tularemia, dubbed the "first American disease" because the bacterium was first identified in McCoy's lab in California, and was then the most celebrated bacteriologist in America.* If anyone could solve the outbreak, Cumming figured, it was McCoy. But when McCoy read Martin's telegram he could not help smiling. *Parrot fever?* It sounded like the sort of diagnosis you might encounter in the medical columns of the yellow press or a joke in the funny pages. Certainly, McCoy had never heard of parrot fever. But then McCoy was a busy man—America was in the grip of an influenza epidemic, a recrudescence, it was feared, of the Spanish flu, and he and his deputy, Charlie Armstrong, were working day and night on a serum for postvaccinal encephalitis, a "sleeping sickness" that affected some individuals who'd received the smallpox vaccine. Nevertheless, McCoy thought it best to check with his colleague.

"Armstrong, what do *you* know about parrot fever," McCoy demanded. "What do I know about it? I don't know a *thing* about it," Armstrong admitted.

Within days, however, McCoy and Armstrong would come to rue their ignorance as one by one laboratory workers tasked with investigating whether parrots were implicated in the outbreaks seen in Annapolis and elsewhere, fell ill. Indeed, by February Armstrong and several other personnel at the "Hygienic," as the ramshackle red-brick

---

* McCoy first isolated the bacterium of tularemia in 1911 while examining squirrels for plague lesions in Tulare County, California. Transmitted by ticks, mites, and lice, tularemia is endemic to every state in the US, the principal reservoirs being wild rabbits and deer. In humans, the tick or deer fly bites can result in ulceration and swelling of the lymph glands; hence its confusion with plague.

laboratory overlooking the Potomac was known, had been removed to the nearby US Naval Hospital. By the time the outbreak concluded in March, Armstrong's longtime assistant, Henry "Shorty" Anderson, was dead. In the end, it fell to McCoy to conduct the critical passage experiments on parrots in the basement of the Hygienic in an attempt to isolate the "virus" of psittacosis and develop a serum. But the tests were inconclusive and in the end McCoy had been forced to chloroform the birds and fumigate the Hygienic from top to bottom to prevent the putative virus from escaping the building. As the science writer Paul de Kruif put it in his book *Men Against Death*, McCoy "never smiled nor even muttered" as he performed this grim task, "but just killed and killed and at the end of it swashed out every last cage with creosol, and gave all the dead bodies of those assorted unhappy experimental creatures a decent and thorough burning in the laboratory incinerator."

TODAY FEW PEOPLE recall the hysteria surrounding the great parrot fever pandemic of 1929–1930, but in an era when parrots were all the rage and itinerant peddlers went door-to-door with "lovebirds" for widows and bored housewives, the idea that one's pet parrot or parakeet might be harboring a deadly pathogen from the Amazon was the stuff of domestic nightmares and a story few newspaper editors could resist. Indeed, were it not for the yellow press, and the Hearst newspaper group in particular, it is unlikely that the connection between parrots and psittacosis would have come to light so fast, or that the PHS would have reacted so quickly. The story about the Argentine theatrical troupe had appeared in the January 5 edition of the *American Weekly*, a lavish supplement distributed with the Sunday editions of the *New York American* and other papers in the Hearst group, under the headline "Killed by a Pet Parrot." Mrs. Martin probably read the story in the *Baltimore American* sandwiched between an article about a tony twice-divorced couple and the "astonishing confessions" of a slave trader. Morrill Goddard, the editor of the *American Weekly*, had spotted the tale about the troupe in an obscure Argentine scientific journal the previous November and had wired the paper's Buenos Aires correspondent, asking for further details. The correspondent found the theater where the troupe had been performing shuttered, but managed to trace the surviving cast members. The most prominent victim had been Carmen Mas, the show's star and a well-known Argentinian comedian. Her leading man, Florencia Paravincini, had also been felled by the disease, but, according to the Hearst correspondent, after "17 days of agony" had recovered. Nevertheless the "bacillus passed from the parrot" had exacted a considerable toll. Prior to the attack Paravincini had been a "big, heavy-set man with hair as black as leather." Now, he weighed less than one hundred pounds and his hair was "as white as snow." It was a doctor at the hospital who had put two and two together. After speaking to the company's prop man, he learned that the actors had been required to pet the parrot on stage and that said bird had since died. As a result, an alert was issued by the *Asistencia Publica*, the Argentine National Health Board, and soon reports of similar outbreaks connected to sickly parrots but wrongly diagnosed as typhoid or influenza were coming to light. In Cordoba, fifty cases were traced to a parrot dealer who had set up shop in a local boarding house. His birds were promptly slaughtered but too late to prevent the distribution of other suspect psittacines. According to the correspondent, the outbreaks in Argentina were entirely avoidable and would not have occurred had dealers observed some simple precautions familiar to indigenous forest peoples accustomed to living alongside wild birds in their natural habitat.

> In semitropical parts of Argentina where the parrots are caught,
> the parrot disease is well known among the natives, who never
> have the creatures for pets, and keep away from them unless

they make a business of catching and shipping them to the cities. The professional parrot catcher takes care not to get hold of a sick bird. If by mistake he does catch a "quiet one" he knows it is deadly and lets it go as well as any healthy captives with which it may have come in contact.

The outbreak in Cordoba was subsequently traced to a consignment of 5,000 parrots imported from Brazil that had been kept in unsanitary conditions in overcrowded crates. By the time Goddard came to learn of the outbreaks, the connection between psittacosis and Brazilian parrots was well known in Argentina and the authorities had outlawed the trade. However, passengers on cruise ships calling at Buenos Aires were largely ignorant of the ban, creating an opening for unscrupulous dealers to offload their sickly birds on unsuspecting tourists. It was this practice that most likely led to the introduction of psittacosis to the United States.

As the term *pandemic* implies, the United States was not the only country affected. In the summer of 1929, four cases of suspected psittacosis were reported in Birmingham, England, and by March of the following year one hundred cases had been recorded across England and Wales. One notable early victim was a ship's carpenter who had purchased two parrots in Buenos Aires, only to see them perish on the voyage to London (when he presented at the London Hospital in December 1929, the carpenter's symptoms were mistaken for typhoid, just as with the Kalmeys in Annapolis). Although most cases seemed to involve sustained exposure to live birds, British researchers observed that this was not always the case, one example being a man who had merely stopped for a beer in a public house in which a sick parrot had been present. By January 1930, similar outbreaks were also being reported in Germany, Italy, Switzerland, France, Denmark, Algeria, Holland, and Egypt. There were even reports of an outbreak in Honolulu.

During the first week of illness, most patients appeared comparatively well in spite of running high temperatures. After five or six days,
however, headache, insomnia, and an irritable cough would set in, and
they would complain of profound exhaustion, their symptoms often
being accompanied by lung consolidation. Soon after, many patients
slipped into delirium and became semicomatose. This was the critical period, with death often following soon after. However, in other
cases, just as it looked as if the illness was about to take a fatal turn,
the patient's temperature would fall and his condition would suddenly
improve. Full recovery might take a further week or two, and sometimes as long as eight. During this protracted convalescence period,
physicians had to constantly monitor their patients' temperatures, as
relapses were frequent.

It was not until much later, of course, that doctors would become
familiar with the typical course of the illness and recognize it as psittacosis. Instead, it was the story in the *American Weekly* and Dr. Martin's telegram that appears to have alerted Cumming to the outbreak
and prompted him to put McCoy and Armstrong onto the case. By
then, psittacosis was widely seeded in cities on the eastern seaboard
of the United States and had already been communicated via dealers
to other caged birds popular with American consumers, such as shell
parakeets (Australian budgerigars). The result was that as parrot fever
spread from Annapolis, to Baltimore, New York, and Los Angeles, the
outbreak became a headline writer's dream. "Parrot Fever Hits Trio at
Annapolis," declared the *Washington Post* on its front page on January 8, 1930. "Parrot Disease Fatal to Seven," reported the *Los Angeles
Times* three days later. "Women's Case Brings Parrot Victims to 19,"
announced the *Baltimore Sun* on January 16.

For widows and bored housewives, caged birds were the FM radios
of their day. The chirping of canaries provided a soothing background
music, punctuating the drudgery of household tasks, and, in the case
of parakeets—parrots' smaller, sprightlier cousin—their facility for

words and humorous phrases provided a facsimile of human conversation. Estimating that New York City alone was home to some 30,000 parrots, *National Geographic* dubbed Amazons and African grays "the ballyhoo barkers of birdom, noisy clever, side-show performers of the tropical forest rainforest." Their pint-sized cousin, the lovebird (genus *Agapornis*), had a reputation for similarly buffoonish behavior, and with their talent for hanging upside down or dancing on their owners' shoulders were a source of endless amusement for children and an entertainment for house guests. Little wonder then that in 1929 nearly 50,000 parrots, parakeets, and lovebirds, and some 500,000 canaries were imported to the United States. These birds arrived not only from Brazil and Argentina, but from Colombia, Cuba, Trinidad, Salvador, Mexico, and Japan. The majority entered the United States via New York, the center of the East Coast bird trade. However, in the case of Australian budgerigars, the main ports of entry were San Francisco and Los Angeles. Indeed, following the Wall Street crash in 1929, a huge bird breeding industry had grown up in Southern California, with hundreds of independent breeders raising lovebirds in their backyards to supplement their incomes. To the naked eye these birds appeared perfectly healthy. However, when they were packed into crowded aviaries or containers and shipped across state lines, many began to shed the virus and transmit the infection. It would prove an invisible and combustible combination.

DESPITE ITS NAME, parrot fever or psittacosis is not confined only to parrotlike birds but has been isolated from some 450 other bird species, including canaries, finches, pigeons, doves, and kestrels.* Moreover, although human infections are typically acquired by exposure to parakeets, bird-to-human transmission has also been documented from

* In nonpsittacine birds, the infection is known as ornithosis.

poultry and free-ranging birds. The culprit is a tiny intracellular parasite, *Chlamydophila psittaci*, a member of the same family of bacteria that transmits chlamydia, a common infection of the eye and genital tract. In the wild, psittacosis lives in equilibrium with its host. Hatchlings are usually infected in the nest through contact with mature birds who harbor the bacillus in their guts. Under natural conditions this contact results in a mild infection that confers lifelong immunity. However, under conditions of stress, such as when food becomes scarce or birds are packed into small crates or confined to cages for long periods, immunity can wane and the infection can be reignited. Typically, a bird's feathers become rough and dirty, and instead of squawking and clawing at the bars of the cage it becomes listless and inert. Sometimes, bloody fluid may leak from its beak and nose, but the most common symptom is diarrhea. It is the feces that pose the principal threat to humans, especially when they become dry and powdery, as occurs in cool conditions. Then, all it takes is a flap of the birds' wings or a sudden breeze from an open window for the particles to be wafted into the atmosphere. The final stage comes when a person enters the same space and inhales the aerosolized particles, allowing the psittacosis bacillus to lodge in the respiratory tract from where it is free to colonize the lungs. Sickness usually occurs six to ten days later, the first sign being a fever accompanied by headache, an irritable dry cough and, on occasion, discharges of bloody mucus from the nose.

It is likely that aboriginal peoples from South America suffered psittacosis from time to time, particularly given the fondness of the Awa and other Brazilian tribes for headdresses featuring brightly colored feathers from macaws, parrots, and toucans. However, it is unlikely that they would have noticed sudden die-offs due to epizootics, since birds falling from the trees in the jungle would have been camouflaged by vegetable debris on the forest floor or rapidly consumed by insects and other scavengers. By contrast, sudden die-offs of birds in captivity are highly visible and difficult to ignore.

No doubt European aristocrats who started the vogue for importing exotic birds from Africa and elsewhere noted such occurrences as early as the eighteenth century, but it was not until 1872 that Jakob Ritter, a Swiss physician living in Ulster, near Zurich, gave the first detailed description of the disease when an outbreak occurred at his brother's house, infecting seven people and killing three. Ritter named the disease "pneumotyphus" and blamed it on a consignment of parrots and finches caged in his brother's study that had recently been imported from Hamburg. This was followed, in 1882, by a second outbreak in Switzerland, this time in Bern, in which two people died. On that occasion, suspicion fell on some sick parrots imported from London. However, the outbreak that attracted widest comment occurred in Paris in 1892 and centered on the homes of two bird fanciers who had recently shipped some five hundred parrots to the French capital from Buenos Aires. During the sea crossing, three hundred birds had died, and people coming into contact with the survivors had rapidly developed symptoms of influenza. On this occasion the outbreak had a mortality rate of 33 percent, prompting the interest of Edmond Nocard, a young assistant of Pasteur. Nocard was unable to get hold of any live birds implicated in the outbreak. Instead, he examined a packet of dried wings taken from parrots that had died during the voyage. From their bone marrow, he was able to cultivate a small Gram-negative bacterium. He then injected or fed the organism to a wide variety of test animals—parrots, pigeons, mice, rabbits and guinea pigs—and demonstrated that in all cases it caused a fatal illness similar to the human disease. Nocard named the microbe *Bacillus psittacosis*, psittacosis being the Greek word for parrot. However, other researchers found it difficult to cultivate Nocard's bacillus from the blood, lungs, urine, or feces of presumed human cases, and as agglutination tests proved similarly negative or inconsistent, doubts gradually grew as to the bacillus's etiological role.

Scientists were right to question Nocard's claim: in fact, the organism he had isolated was a type of salmonella and had nothing to do with psittacosis. Unfortunately, this would not become known until after the 1929–1930 outbreak. In the meantime, just as with Pfeiffer's erroneous claim about the bacterial etiology of influenza, Nocard's error spread confusion, making medics and public health officials reluctant to accept that parrots had anything to do with the human cases of typhoid-like illness.* This only compounded the uncertainty and fears about the source of the epidemic.

Scientists were not the only ones to fail the public. Reflecting on the parrot fever pandemic in 1933 in his best-selling book, *Men Against Death*, Paul de Kruif would describe the outbreak and the panic that accompanied it as "one of our American hysterias." If so it was a hysteria that he and other journalists helped engender. This was a pity, as de Kruif ought to have known better. Before turning to science writing de Kruif had worked as a bacteriologist at the University of Michigan and during the First World War had served as a captain in the US Sanitary Corps, where he helped develop an antitoxin for gas gangrene. Afterwards, he joined the Rockefeller Institute, but just as it looked as if he were set for an illustrious career as a medical researcher, de Kruif wrote an ill-advised book, *Our Medicine Men* (1922), containing thinly disguised portraits of his Rockefeller colleagues. The book cost him his position at the Rockefeller Institute but launched his career as a science journalist. In 1925, he teamed up with Sinclair Lewis to write *Arrowsmith*, a runaway best seller about a country doctor turned research scientist that fired the imaginations of a generation of American medical researchers. This was followed in 1926 by *Microbe Hunters*, a nonfiction book profiling the pioneers of microbiology, such as Koch, Pasteur, and the Nobel Prize–winning

---

* The ease with which people contracted psittacosis in the presence of parrots was seen as further evidence that the infective agent must be an intestinal parasite, even though in many cases patients had not touched sick birds or handled their fecal matter but had merely been in the same room as them.

physiologist Paul Ehrlich, who had reversed centuries of medical superstition by applying laboratory techniques to the study of infectious disease. But successful as these books were, de Kruif's bread and butter was "scare" stories about obscure microorganisms that posed a theoretical threat to American housewives. "In American milk today there lurks a terrible, wasting fever, that may keep you in bed for a couple of weeks, that may fasten itself on you for one, or for two, or even for seven years—that might culminate by killing you," he informed the readers of *Ladies Home Journal* in 1929. De Kruif was referring to undulant fever, or brucellosis, a disease of cattle that, while it might cause cows to abort prematurely, in truth posed little threat to people. However, in an era before pasteurization when many housewives still drank "raw" milk drawn from local dairy herds, undulant fever was a perfect candidate for a germ panic, fitting the template of what medical historian Nancy Tomes calls the "killer germ genre of journalism." Drawing on the latest microbiological discoveries and Progressive Era messages about the importance of sanitation and personal hygiene, this genre played on the dangers that lurked in everyday objects, such as coins, library books, or drinking cups. Dust and insects were targets of similar scaremongering, hence the advertisements urging housewives to mop regularly with disinfectants and spray their homes with insecticides. By the 1920s, as Americans adopted new germ-conscious regimes, even handshaking and kissing babies came to be frowned upon.

These fears were not only used to sell bleaches, detergents, and bug sprays, they were also a way of selling newspapers; hence Goddard's decision to hype the story about the Argentine theatrical troupe. In a germophobic era, even the normally level-headed *New York Times* was not immune to the parrot panic. "Many have long had the feeling that there is something diabolical about the parrot tribe," opined a columnist at the height of the scare. "More than one family pet, known by its owners to possess the amiable and gentle disposition of a kitten, is regarded with fear and trembling by visitors. Until more has been learned about the nature of the malady the safest course seems absolute ostracism for recent immigrants of the parrot family."

Within days of that editorial, however, the *New York Times* was quoting the opinion of a Viennese expert who thought the scare "baseless" and that Americans were victims of "mass suggestion." Two days later, psittacosis—or parrots, at least—had become a laughing matter as the paper regaled its readers with the story of Secretary of State Henry Stimson's pet parrot, "The Old Soak." Stimson's bird had been caught misbehaving while his master was overseas, cursing at tourists and their guides as they entered the Pan-American Building. The bird, apparently, was "quite a linguist," and was said to have learned the profanities "during his days in the Philippines." As a punishment, The Old Soak was confined to the basement of the Pan-American building where he could curse without giving offense. However, no joking could hide the fact that America's microbe hunters had missed something that had been known to their medical colleagues in Argentina since the previous summer, and that had most likely been incubating under their noses since the fall of 1929. How had this been possible, and who would be the person to restore the reputation of the US Public Health Service?

CHARLIE ARMSTRONG is a type that has almost disappeared from American medicine today: a scientist equally at home in the laboratory and the field, who combined serious medical research with a career devoted to fighting infectious disease and improving public health. A graduate of Johns Hopkins Medical School, Armstrong's interest in public health was fired by his early experiences as medical officer in the US Marine Hospital Service on Ellis Island in 1916, where it was his job to examine immigrants suspected of introducing diseases like trachoma and typhus to the United States. Two years later, as an assistant surgeon on the *Seneca*, a US coast guard cutter on escort duty in the Atlantic, he had witnessed the first wave of Spanish flu when an outbreak occurred on his boat off the coast of Gibraltar, prompting him to hoist the yellow quarantine ensign. Later, while serving at the Fore River Shipyard, near Boston, Armstrong had also treated sailors affected by the deadly second wave. It was an experience he would never forget. Asked years later what the flu was like, he told a reporter: "with influenza you think you are going to die and afraid that you won't." After the war, Armstrong was posted to the Ohio Department of Health, where he continued his investigations into influenza and honed his epidemiological skills. Then, in 1921, he was posted to the Hygienic. He would remain there until his retirement in 1950, a period in which he would also contract malaria, dengue fever, encephalitis, Q fever, and tularemia. Despite the risks that his laboratory work exposed him to, however, Armstrong was a tireless investigator. His most notable contribution to scientific research came in 1934 when he isolated a new neurotropic virus—a virus with affinity for nerve tissue, which he named *lymphocytic choriomeningitis*, from the spinal fluid of monkeys artificially infected with material from the 1933 St. Louis encephalitis epidemic. This was followed, in 1940, by the first transmission of a polio virus from monkeys to rats and mice, an experimental innovation that laid the ground for subsequent investigations into the immunology of the disease and the development of human polio vaccines. Awarded the Sedgwick Memorial Medal of the American Public Health Association the following year, Armstrong was hailed as someone who had made "a distinct contribution to the knowledge of every disease with which he has worked." In short, he was the epitome of the male microbe hunter. As de Kruif put it, Armstrong was "thick set, with reddish hair and round china-blue eyes set wide apart in a face that couldn't keep from smiling," and definitely not the sort of man who would "own a parrot let alone kiss it." In spite of his skepticism about parrot fever, however, when

McCoy summoned him to his office, Armstrong immediately agreed to drop his vaccine experiments and travel to Annapolis to see if there was any truth in the rumor.

According to de Kruif, by now requests for information about the mysterious new disease were pouring into Washington, and Cumming's desk was piled with "stacks of yellow and blue slips." For once, de Kruif was not exaggerating. In her history of the PHS, Bess Furman reports that by early January thirty-six cases of suspected psittacosis had been reported to the surgeon general, and his desk was "deluged" with urgent telegrams. Like all good disease detectives, Armstrong headed to the scene of the crime: Lillian's bedside. Her pet parrot had long been buried but she still had the cage and, miraculously, it still contained some of the bird's droppings. Following protocol, Armstrong shared some of the cleanings from the cage with William Royal Stokes, the head of bacteriology at the Baltimore Department of Health, so that he could conduct independent tests. Before returning to Washington, Armstrong warned Stokes to be careful when culturing organisms from the material, reminding him that many people suspected that psittacosis "might be a virus," not a bacterium. Stokes promised to heed Armstrong's warning, but within a matter of weeks he would be dead.

By January 8, 1930, Lillian and her son and daughter-in-law were not the only ones thought to have parrot fever. Four employees of the pet store at North Eutaw Street were also ill, as was a woman who had bought a parrot at another store in southeast Baltimore. Then, on January 10, came the fatalities. The first victim was a Baltimore woman, Mrs. Louise Schaeffer, whose death had originally been attributed to pneumonia; it was only when Baltimore health officials questioned her family that it emerged she had been in contact with a parrot several days earlier. However, it was the second death that really alarmed health officials because it occurred in Toledo, Ohio, nearly five hundred miles to the northwest of Baltimore. The victim was Mrs. Percy

Q. Williams. She had died at Toledo's Mercy Hospital three weeks after her husband had returned from Cuba with a gift of three parrots (one of the parrots had died shortly after his return). It was the first indication of the true extent of the epidemic and the challenge facing state and federal health officials. Cumming had previously avoided making a public statement. Now he had no choice. He "did not fear an epidemic," he said, as it was generally believed that psittacosis was transmitted "only from bird to human being, and not from person to person." Nevertheless, he advised Americans to avoid handling recently imported parrots until the completion of Armstrong's investigation. "There is at present no indication of widespread prevalence of the disease, but I would urge that people avoid contact with possible conveyors, the birds."

Cumming's statement was all that newspapers needed to run with the story. Even the *New York Times* displayed the reports prominently. "Parrot Fever Kills 2 In This Country," it declared on January 11, placing the story at the top of page 3. "Woman in Baltimore and Another in Toledo are Victims of Rare Disease. Eleven others are ill," continued the subhead. The following day, with reports of further suspect cases in Ohio involving several clerks in the poultry department of a Toledo store, the *New York Times* promoted the story to page one. "Hunts For Source of 'Parrot Fever,'" it declared, above a report describing the efforts of Baltimore state health officials and the Bureau of Animal Industry and Biological Survey to confirm the source of the parrots sold in Baltimore pet shops. "We do not consider it practical to place an embargo on importation before making sure where the sick parrots are coming from," stated Cumming in a game attempt to reassure an increasingly nervous public.

By the middle of January, Baltimore officials working with colleagues from the state health department had visited seven pet stores in the city and the homes of thirty-eight people who had recently purchased parrots. Of these, thirty-six were ill with the same symptoms as the Kalmeys. This so alarmed Daniel S. Hatfield, the director of the Bureau of Communicable Diseases, that he ordered an immediate moratorium on the sale of parrots and the isolation of all birds seized in Baltimore pet stores. However, Hatfield was not so cautious when it came to protecting his own health, and on January 19, while assisting Stokes, he contracted psittacosis and was rushed to Baltimore's Mercy Hospital. Hatfield was lucky. Unlike Stokes, who by now was autopsying parrots daily and, presumably, exposing himself to massive amounts of virus, he had a mild case of the disease and survived.

If there was any doubt before about the role of foreign birds, the Baltimore investigations dispelled them: out of the seven pet shops investigated, four were shown to be the source of diseased parrots. Nearly all were traced to shipments from Central or South America that had come via dealers in New York. If that was the case, it was highly likely that those same dealers had sold diseased birds to pet stores in other cities. Sure enough, when Armstrong wired public health officials across the country he was inundated with information, and birds, both dead and alive, began arriving from Baltimore, Maine, Chicago, New Haven, and Los Angeles. And as more and more cases came to light, so the death toll crept up. Women, many of them widows, constituted the majority of victims, most likely because they were the principal recipients of lovebirds. Peddlers usually sold the birds singly to facilitate their bonding with their owners. Women were also most likely to kiss the birds affectionately, or care for them when they fell sick. By the final week in January, more than fifty cases had been reported nationwide, including fourteen in New York, where, under pressure from the city's health commissioner, bird dealers were forced to accept a voluntary embargo. Soon, orphaned birds began turning up all over the city, including in the vestibule of a house in East Elmhurst, Queens. Taking pity on the young foundling, which had a chipped beak, the householder turned it over to the Society for the Prevention of Cruelty to Animals. "Fear of psittacosis," reported the *New York Times*, "is thought to be the reason for the abandonment of the bird."

At this point, the only persons interested in collecting parrots were Armstrong and his assistant, "Shorty" Anderson (so called because he stood just five feet six inches tall). By January 16, Armstrong and Anderson had everything they needed to conduct bacteriological tests: parrots both dead and alive, the scrapings from Lillian's birdcage, and blood from human patients. Well aware that the birds were highly contagious and that they were probably dealing with a "filter-passing" virus, Armstrong decided to confine the experiments to two small dark rooms in the basement of the Hygienic. According to de Kruif, these rooms were "dank, frowsty little holes hardly bigger than coal bins, [and] an insult to offer to any self-respecting microbe hunter for a laboratory." Worse, the healthy birds were "clawing green devils," who were constantly scrabbling to escape their cages or scattering food and fecal droppings onto the floor. To try to contain them, Armstrong and Anderson placed the most violent birds in cages they'd rigged from metal garbage cans enclosed with wire mesh covers. In addition, they kept the birds behind moist curtains soaked in disinfectant and put troughs containing creosol in the doorways. They also periodically scrubbed the walls with disinfectant and wore heavy rubber gloves and aprons when extracting birds from their cages. Nevertheless, de Kruif considered the Hygienic one of the most "odiferously untidy" buildings he had ever visited. The Rockefeller virologist, Thomas Rivers, a leading authority on filterable viruses, concurred, remarking that the only thing hygienic about the building was its name.

Despite this unpromising working environment, however, within days Armstrong had succeeded in communicating the disease from sick to healthy birds using either the droppings from infected birds or ground-up tissue from a dead parrot (according to de Kruif, the deceased bird came from Stokes in Baltimore). Armstrong also

observed that while some of the sick birds died, many survived inoculation with infective material, after which they became asymptomatic carriers.* According to de Kruif, Anderson was particularly adept
at grabbing the parrots without getting "gaffed" by them. Just days
before, both men had considered themselves "parrot ignoramuses."
Now, "by a little jab of next to nothing through a needle," the birds
were sitting hunched in their cages "with their heads bent forward,"
and Armstrong and Anderson had the feeling they were "getting control of this weird disease." Try as they might, however, they could not
isolate the bacillus described by Nocard, or culture any other organism from the ground-up material. It seemed increasingly likely that
psittacosis was a filter-passer that could only be transmitted from bird
to bird or from bird to human by close contact. But how precisely the
virus was conveyed from parrots and whether people were also capable
of transmitting it independently of birds, was anyone's guess. Perhaps
patients communicated the virus via the respiratory route when they
coughed infectious material? If that was the case, it might become as
transmissible as flu. Clearly, it was imperative to make a serum before
the unthinkable happened and psittacosis became a true pandemic.

Armstrong would need that serum sooner than he anticipated.
Based on the initial results of his investigation, on January 24 President
Herbert Hoover issued an Executive Order prohibiting "the immediate importation of parrots into the United States, its possessions and
dependencies from any foreign port" until such time as the causative
organism and its means of transmission could be ascertained. Unfortunately, when Armstrong strode into the "old red brick building on
the hill" to resume the investigation the following morning he found
Shorty slumped over his desk, complaining of a high fever and a "rot-

---

* This was an important clue to the natural history of the disease, one that helped
explain why wild birds were not continually dropping dead of psittacosis and epizootics were rare. However, the significance of the finding would only become apparent
to researchers in the mid-1930s. See discussion below.

ten headache." Normally, when work was going well Shorty was "all smiles and cheerful profanity." A born "lab-swipe," Shorty was never happier than when he was microbe-hunting, claimed de Kruif. "Now he looked awful." It was not difficult to diagnose the cause of his malaise. Armstrong arranged for him to be admitted to the US Naval Hospital, where X-rays showed a sinister cloud at the base of his left lung. It was at this point that McCoy stepped in and, over the objections of his employees and family, joined Armstrong in the basement. As McCoy tried to mimic Shorty's technique of gaffing the birds, Armstrong rushed back and forth between the laboratory and the hospital to check on his assistant's condition. There was little sign of improvement, and in desperation Armstrong drew blood from Shorty's veins and collected expectorations from his bedsheets in order to inoculate the fluids into parrots and other test animals. At the same time, to see how parrots became infected, he and McCoy also placed parts of dead parrots in cages along with healthy birds. Armstrong may have thought that by co-opting Shorty into the experiments, he would buy his assistant some more time. But though he was able to confirm that psittacosis was a filter passer, he could not forestall the inevitable and on February 8 Shorty died. Scrupulous about paying his bills, his last request was that Armstrong settle his outstanding debts.

Unfortunately, it was a request Armstrong was unable to honor as that very day he was also admitted to the hospital. As Shorty was laid to rest in Arlington National Cemetery with full military honors (he was an ex-navy man), Armstrong's temperature spiked from 102° to 104° F. The following day, an X-ray showed a white shadow enveloping his left lung, confirmation that he had pneumonia and was almost certainly infected with the same bug. When McCoy saw the X-ray he decided to take a gamble by using a method of unknown and questionable value: namely, the administration of convalescent blood serum. It had been known since the 1890s that survivors of diphtheria and other bacterial diseases were immune to reinfection, and that their immunity was associated with antibodies circulating in their blood. More-over, if their blood was purified and the antibodies separated from the red corpuscles, the resulting serum could also be used to protect immune-naïve individuals from the same diseases. By the 1920s, this principle was also being applied to viral diseases, such as influenza and polio, but although the transfer of passive serum from survivors of flu and polio sometimes appeared to confer protection, it was far from clear if this protection was due to the serum or some other factor. Moreover, since there was no way of screening blood for impurities in the 1920s, physicians had no way of knowing whether or not passive serums contained active viral material or some other undiscovered virus, such as hepatitis. Ironically, one of the biggest serum skeptics of all was McCoy. Hardly a month went by without a claim from some fly-by-night pharmaceutical firm that it had developed a serum for pneumonia or meningitis. As the head of the Hygienic, it was McCoy's job to examine these requests and deny licenses to those he considered questionable. Now, he threw caution to the wind and instructed Roscoe Spencer of the Rocky Mountain Laboratory to head the search for potential serum donors. Spencer had recently developed a vaccine against spotted fever, a tick-borne disease endemic to Montana and some midwestern states—an endeavor for which he would be awarded the gold medal of the American Medical Association—and was quite happy to turn errand boy to help a fellow microbiologist stricken in the line of duty. According to de Kruif, the serum came from an elderly Maryland lady who graciously refused payment for her blood. Others report Spencer procured the precious serum from a physician at Johns Hopkins Hospital in Baltimore. What is not in dispute is that within hours of the serum entering his veins, Armstrong rallied and his condition improved.

Over the next two weeks, as Armstrong grew stronger, McCoy continued his investigation, mashing up the livers and spleens of dead parakeets before passing them through filters and inoculating the filtrate into healthy birds. Fearing further infections, McCoy forbade his staff from entering the makeshift laboratory in the basement of the north building of the Hygienic Laboratory, and from February 7 insisted on conducting the autopsies of parrots and disposing of their carcasses in person. At this point, it was still not known whether psittacosis could be communicated from person to person or whether the microbe was also conveyed as an aerosol in dust particles. To minimize the risk of accidental contamination, the only person McCoy allowed to approach the basement laboratory was the general foreman whose job it was to bring sandwiches for McCoy and feed for the birds. He usually handed these items to McCoy at the threshold and did not enter the rooms himself. To reduce the chances of the sick birds accidentally spreading the infection to healthy parrots, McCoy also strung a muslin curtain across the archway between the laboratory rooms and wetted the floor each morning with creosol. Nevertheless, on occasion, McCoy would find diseased parrots, who had somehow freed themselves from the cages, wandering in a room reserved for healthy birds.

Despite these precautions, within eight days of Armstrong's illness several other staff at the Hygienic had also fallen ill. The first casualty was the north building's night watchman, Robert Lanham, who came on duty at midnight and left every morning at 8 a.m., a period when laboratory work was suspended and no autopsies were being carried out. Lanham's only risk was that he had briefly been in the same room as Anderson on January 27, the day Shorty fell ill. However, Lanham had fallen sick eighteen days later, which was well outside the presumed incubation period.

The next person to contract psittacosis was a laboratory assistant, whose symptoms became apparent on February 28. Unlike Lanham, she had never breathed the same air as someone incubating psittacosis. However, her office was next door to the basement room where McCoy kept the healthy birds, and she had also handled material for culturing the organism, though since her principal role was to look for salmonella and streptococci McCoy thought it unlikely that she could have been exposed to psittacosis this way. However, the next group of casualties left McCoy in no doubt that his precautions had failed and that the north building was thoroughly contaminated. The first to fall ill was a medical officer whose office was on the side of the corridor opposite the autopsy room. The next day, March 11, the general foreman was also taken ill, followed in quick succession by two cleaners and two bacteriologists engaged in research on other diseases. Except for McCoy, no one escaped the disease. Even Ludvig Hektoen, a distinguished pathologist and chairman of the National Research Council, who was doing private research at the Hygienic and had merely spent his afternoons in one of the rooms, was admitted to the hospital.

All told, between January 25 and March 15, eleven people at the Hygienic were hospitalized with psittacosis. Despite drawing a floor plan of the infections, McCoy could discern no pattern in the cases, leading him to speculate that psittacosis may have been transferred to the upper floors by mice or cockroaches. The other possibility, of course, was that the organism had been aerosolized and the building was full of infectious fomites. Either way, drastic action was needed. So it was that on March 15 McCoy ordered everyone to evacuate the building and shut the laboratory. Experimental animals not involved in psittacosis research were removed to temporary lodgings. Then McCoy entered the basement for the last time and exterminated all those that remained—a menagerie of parrots, guinea pigs, mice, rats, pigeons, and monkeys. Next, he burned their bodies in the incinerator and scrubbed their cages with creosol, and methodically worked his way through the building to seal the windows on each floor. Finally, when he was sure there was no living thing left inside the Hygienic, he ordered a fumigation squad to blitz the building with cyanide. The legend goes that so much gas was used that sparrows flying fifty feet above the Hygienic stopped in mid-flight and plummeted to Earth.

The next day, the headline in the Sunday edition of the *Washington Post* read, "Parrot Fever Panic Seizes Laboratory."

McCoy was not the only one panicking. By now, Roscoe Spencer was rushing up and down the East Coast in search of serum. The flasks of blood he brought back to Washington were used to treat the Hygienic personnel, and by April all the building's staff had recovered, Armstrong included. Others were not so fortunate, however. Stokes got two transfusions of Roscoe's serum but died on February 9, the day after Anderson. For those stricken with psittacosis there was good reason to be afraid. The infection often proved fatal, with thirty-three deaths recorded in the United States between November 1929 and May 1930. Of the 167 cases where the sex of the victim was known, 105, or two-thirds, had been women. Another badly affected country was Germany, with 215 cases and 45 deaths. Indeed, at one point Berlin Zoo had been forced to bar its gates to frightened parrot owners desperately looking for a temporary refuge for their birds. In all, some fifteen countries were affected. By the time the pandemic ended in May 1930, eight hundred cases had been recorded worldwide, with an average mortality rate of 15 percent.

Armstrong and McCoy were not the only researchers puzzled by the sudden appearance of psittacosis and the failure to find Nocard's bacillus. Soon, researchers in other countries were also convinced the pathogen must be a filter passer and that Nocard had mistaken it for salmonella, the bacterium that causes typhoid. The first to succeed was a team led by Samuel Bedson, a senior researcher at the London Hospital. Taking parrots associated with human cases, Bedson and his colleagues emulsified the dead birds' liver and spleen, passed the material through a Chamberland filter, and then inoculated budgerigars with the filtrate. The budgerigars died within five days. Next, Bedson's group showed that by passaging filtered material from diseased budgerigars every few days, the organism gradually lost its virulence. Bedson's conclusion was unequivocal: "the aetiological agent of psittacosis in parrots is a virus which cannot be cultivated on ordinary bacteriological media, and which is capable of passing through some of the more porous filters."

Soon after, Charles Krumwiede, a researcher at the New York Board of Health, demonstrated that the virus could be readily transferred from parakeets to white mice. This greatly facilitated laboratory study of psittacosis as white mice were far less infectious than birds. Nevertheless, Krumwiede was forced to suspend his studies when he fell ill, resulting in his research being taken up by Thomas Rivers. Aware that psittacosis was highly infectious, the Rockefeller researcher left nothing to chance, insisting that his team wear full body suits, with glass goggles in the helmets and rubber gloves attached to the sleeves— precautions that foreshadowed measures that would become standard in Biosafety Level Four laboratories used to study Ebola and other hazardous pathogens sixty years later. Rivers also demonstrated that psittacosis could be transferred to rabbits, guinea pigs, and monkeys. However, in monkeys the infectious material only produced typical pneumonia if introduced via the trachea. To Rivers, this suggested that the principal transmission route in humans was via the respiratory tract, not through scratches or parrot bites—a view soon adopted by other researchers.

Although psittacosis was beyond the magnification range of optical microscopes at that time, by now Walter Levinthal of the Robert Koch Institute in Dahlem, Germany, A. C. Coles of the Lister Institute in London, and Ralph Lillie at the Hygienic Laboratory, were reporting distinctive clusters of inclusion bodies in the cytoplasm of patients who had died of psittacosis. Dubbed "Levinthal-Coles-Lillie" or "LCL" bodies, these *could be* observed through an ordinary optical microscope, where they appeared as microcolonies on the surface of the cell, making the diagnosis of psittacosis and the development of agglutination tests far easier. The only point that remained uncertain was the exact mode of transmission. Handling an ill or dead bird was certainly a risk, but there were also plenty of cases in which patients had merely been in the same room or house as a sick parrot. There were even cases in which people had contracted psittacosis after visiting a pet shop or, in the case of baggage handlers, sharing a railway carriage with a sick bird. This was not a message that pet shop owners or bird breeders wished to hear. On the contrary, many refused to accept that the reports of pneumonia and typhoid-like illness were due to parrots or parakeets at all, much less that psittacosis could be spread via the atmosphere from bird to man. Otherwise, they claimed, breeders and people who worked in pet shops would be ill all the time, but according to dealers the opposite was the case. "So far as it is aware," declared the newly formed Bird Dealers Association of America at a meeting held in New York's Commodore Hotel at the height of the pandemic, "no bird dealers whose hourly contact with feathered pets would render them likely to contract psittacosis if it is communicable to humans, have been affected." Nor could reports of pet owners catching psittacosis directly from imported birds be believed as "any one putting his face near enough a newly imported parrot to catch a disease would sure to be bitten by the untrained bird." In short, the parrot fever "scare" was down to "the active imagination of a Baltimore newspaper man."

One can hardly blame bird dealers for wanting to fight back. America's six leading pet dealers, all of which were based in either New York or Philadelphia, stood to lose $5 million annually from Hoover's import ban. And, in many ways, they were right, for as the panic over imported parrots subsided, foreign birds no longer constituted the principal threat. Instead, it was home-reared birds—parrots and parakeets raised in backyard aviaries—that posed the biggest risk to pet owners, particularly in Southern California where conditions were perfect for breeding birds outdoors year-round. This time it would not be a newspaperman who would spot the danger, however, but a Swiss-trained veterinary pathologist whose laboratory sat

near the summit of a chilly, fog-shrouded hill overlooking the Golden
Gate Bridge.

⌁

IN THE SUMMER OF 1930, while researchers on the East Coast were
developing tools for visualizing psittacosis and refining agglutination
tests, Karl Friedrich Meyer was focused on a mysterious "sleeping
sickness" affecting horses in southern California and other western
states. Educated in Basel and Zurich, Meyer's interest in animal diseases bridged by multiple insect and arthropod vectors was born in
1909 in South Africa, when, as an assistant at Arnold Theiler's (the
father of the Nobel Prize winner Max Theiler) Veterinary Bacteriological Institute in Pretoria, he became the first person to elucidate the life
cycle of the plasmodium of East Coast Fever, a tick-borne disease of
cattle. Soon after, Meyer contracted malaria and was forced to return
to Europe, but he did not stay long. By 1911 he had secured a teaching
position at the University of Pennsylvania's veterinary school. There,
Meyer became acquainted with the leading lights in American pathology and bacteriology, including Theobald Smith, whose groundbreak-
ing study of Texas Cattle Fever was to provoke a rethinking of germ
theory and the role of parasitical infections generally, and Frederick
Novy, the director of the University of Michigan's Hygiene Laboratory,
who had headed the official inquiry into the 1901 bubonic plague outbreak in San Francisco. Through Smith, Meyer was also introduced
to Simon Flexner, the director of the Rockefeller Institute. But rather
than take a job in New York, Meyer decided to head west, lured by the
offer of an assistant professorship at Berkeley and the prospect of a
research position at the newly formed George Williams Hooper Foundation for Medical Research in San Francisco.

Housed in a three-story brick building in the former veterinary
school on Mount Sutro in Parnassus Heights, the Hooper Foundation had been established by Hooper's widow in 1913 with a generous

$1 million bequest and was the first private medical research insti-
tution to be attached to any American university. Although Flexner
warned Meyer that in joining the Hooper, he risked "disappear[ing]
in the Pacific Ocean, because the intelligentsia of the United States
lives within a hundred miles from New York," the Hooper offered
Meyer a degree of intellectual freedom that would have been impossible in the East. Besides, as Meyer acknowledged, he was a "typical Basel squarehead" with a stubborn streak as wide as the Rhine.
In his interactions with colleagues and other scientists, this stub-
bornness could come across as arrogance—an impression not helped
by Meyer's Teutonic bearing, thick German-accented English, and
intolerance of errors, particularly ones that occurred in his laboratory. However, when it came to tracking and identifying the source
of new diseases there was, apparently, no more indefatigable oppo-
nent of microbes. Indeed, in a special tribute published in *Reader's
Digest* in 1950, de Kruif hailed Meyer, then in his 60s, as "the most
versatile microbe hunter since Pasteur." In a career spanning three
decades, Meyer had helped eradicate brucellosis from Californian
dairy herds; had demonstrated that botulism, a deadly food-borne
pathogen, was a highly resistant spore found in soils across America;
and had shown how sylvatic plague was endemic to ground squirrels
and other wild rodent populations across the western United States.
In short, declared de Kruif, Meyer was "an outdoor scientist living in
a state of permanent outdoor emergency . . . [and a] master among
the world's microbe hunters."

History does not record whether Meyer was pleased or embarrassed
by de Kruif's gushing tribute—interviewed in the 1960s, Meyer said
that his former wife suspected de Kruif of trying to "belittle" and
"besmear" him. However, although de Kruif was an alcoholic and
had a turbulent personality, he and Meyer maintained a friendship
for more than three decades, and twice a year de Kruif would make
a point of visiting Meyer in San Francisco, where the pair enjoyed

solitary moments hiking together on Mount Tamalpais, discussing the latest medical breakthroughs, and exchanging gossip about their bacteriological colleagues.

A member of the Sierra Club, Meyer traced his fascination with infectious disease to his boyhood excursions in the Swiss Alps, where he fell into conversation with British climbers recently returned from the plague spots of India; de Kruif was right to link his passion for microbe hunting with his enthusiasm for adventure and outdoor living. So it is little wonder that when reports reached the Hooper of a massive horse epizootic in the San Joaquin Valley, Meyer raced from his laboratory to investigate. There, he found horses wandering aimlessly in circles or listing from side to side. Meyer's veterinary colleagues thought the horses' staggering symptoms were the result of "forage poisoning" due to botulism. However, the San Joaquin epizootic had broken out in June—the wrong time of year for botulism—and vets who visited affected ranches noted that the majority of the victims of "staggers," as the disease was known, were free-ranging horses, not those that had been fed on silage or stacked hay. At autopsy Meyer noted that the horses' brains were inflamed and scarred by microscopic hemorrhages, leading him to suspect that the neurological impairment was caused by a virus. Unfortunately, by the time he came to examine the horses, the virus had disappeared. What Meyer needed was to autopsy the brain of a recently infected horse. His opportunity came later that summer when one of his colleagues located a sick horse on a ranch in Merced. The rancher wanted nothing to do with Meyer's experiment, so Meyer bribed his wife with $20 and, when she signaled that her husband was asleep, snuck into the stable and decapitated the horse in the middle of the night, hottailing it back to San Francisco with its severed head sticking out of the trunk of his car. That very same morning, Meyer extracted the horse's brain, mashed it up, and injected the material into guinea pigs. Soon the guinea pigs' bodies were racked with tremors. Next, they curled up into balls or hunched up like cats, dying four to six days later. After repeating the experiment in rabbits, monkeys, and horses with the same results, Meyer and his colleagues announced that they had isolated a new filter-passing virus. It would be several years before researchers would confirm that, as Meyer had suspected, the virus was a type of encephalitis communicated to horses by mosquitoes breeding in nearby irrigation ditches, and would be able to divine its arboreal life cycle.

Though preoccupied by equine encephalitis, Meyer had followed the parrot fever outbreaks, and Armstrong and McCoy's efforts to passage the virus. However, it was not until the following year that he had reason to initiate his own studies and became interested in the involvement of bird breeders. The impetus came when three elderly women, who had attended a coffee club in Grass Valley in the Sierra Nevadas shortly before Thanksgiving in 1931, died. Local physicians were baffled as to the cause, attributing the women's deaths to, variously, typhoid fever, dysentery, and "toxic pneumonia." However, on reviewing the medical reports and learning that the husband of the woman who had convened the gathering was also ill, Meyer realized that the common denominator was the room where they had gathered. He instructed the local health officer to see if there was a sick or dead parrot there. Meyer's intuition was partially correct: there was no parrot, but on going to the woman's home in Grass Valley the health officer discovered a healthy shell parakeet still in its cage, and another one which had recently died. Meyer immediately ordered the official to disinter the parakeet and send its carcass to the Hooper, together with its live mate. That same evening, at around 10 p.m., Meyer's was astonished to see a driver in a face mask pull up outside his laboratory. It was the official, and on the back seat was the surviving parakeet chirping in its cage. "He was scared out of his wits that he might pick it up," Meyer recalled, "because it was generally known that because it was air-borne this was a highly contagious disease."

To verify his hunch that the bird was infected, Meyer began with a simple exposure test, taking a healthy Japanese ricebird (finch), which he had read was highly susceptible to psittacosis, and placing it in a bell jar with the parakeet. Within two to three weeks the ricebird was dead. The parakeet, meanwhile, appeared "perfectly normal" and continued to shed sufficient virus such that if it was transferred again to a clean bell jar with another ricebird, that bird also became ill and died. When Meyer finally sacrificed the parakeet on January 16, 1932, and inoculated the bird's mashed-up spleen into mice in his laboratory, the mice died within three to four days, suggesting that the "agent was exceedingly virile." To be sure, Meyer repeated the experiment, removing the parakeet from the glass jar every time a finch died and transferring it to a new jar with another finch. After six months, Meyer had his proof: it was the desiccated droppings from the parakeet that were spreading the infection.

In the meantime, in January, the woman's husband had also died. Concerned that there might be a statewide problem, Meyer had pressed the health department to issue a press release. The resulting publicity brought further reports of suspicious deaths involving parakeets from as far south as Tehachapi. Questioning itinerant peddlers who made a living selling parakeets door-to-door, Meyer and his assistant Bernice Eddie discovered that most of the birds had come from backyard aviaries in the Los Angeles area. Many of these breeding establishments belonged to war veterans and had been funded by the bonuses they had received under Depression relief. It was a low-tech and highly profitable business as the birds bred astonishingly fast. All an amateur breeder needed was lumber, wire netting, and a breeding box. Within weeks the pens were full of young hatchlings or "crawlers." These young birds were very popular with pet owners; they could be trained to sit on their fingers and pick seeds. Rather than allow the nestlings to mature, amateur breeders had quickly sold them on to the trade. Indeed, over the Thanksgiving period and in the run-up to

Christmas, Meyer discovered peddlers had crisscrossed the state offering lovebirds as gifts for housewives and widows.

Meyer put out a call to pet shops throughout California requesting that they send him other birds that were visibly sick or were associated with a householder who had recently been hospitalized with psittacosis. Soon, birds were arriving at the Hooper Foundation from as far north as Santa Rosa and as far south as San Luis Obispo. At first glance, the parakeets appeared perfectly healthy, but when Meyer examined their spleens he discovered their organs were swollen and scarred with lesions characteristic of psittacosis. The final proof came when he inoculated mice with the mashed-up bird spleens and the rodents fell ill. The more Meyer and Eddie quizzed peddlers and pet shop owners, the greater became their fear that birds all over California might be harboring these asymptomatic, latent infections. From Pasadena, they obtained twenty-two birds, only to find that nine had enlarged livers and spleens. In some of the breeding pens, Meyer reported, the birds were visibly diseased and "so weak that they were actually crawling on the floor."

Concerned that as many as 40 percent of birds raised in backyard aviaries and professional breeding pens might be carriers of psittacosis, Meyer warned that California could be harboring a huge reservoir of infection. He urged health officials to take action. In particular, he worried that when Californian parakeets were packed into crowded containers and shipped across state lines, the stress caused them to shed the virus, running the risk that they would reignite the epidemic. In other words, Argentine parrots were no longer the main danger: it was Californian birds that now posed the principal threat.

The State Department of Health had previously been blissfully unaware of the extent of California's bird breeding industry and the implications for public health. Now, it declared it was imposing a quarantine and placed an embargo on the transportation of lovebirds across state lines. The measure sparked uproar among California's breeders, particularly as Hoover's embargo on imported parrots the previous year had led to pent-up demand for parakeets, and pet stores in the East were increasingly looking to California to supply the market. Estimates as to the value of this market varied: breeders put it at $5 million; Meyer thought it was worth one-tenth of that. What was not in doubt was that Southern California's temperate year-round Mediterranean climate provided the ideal conditions for bird breeding and that upwards of 3,000 individuals now depended on the trade. What was needed was a system of inspecting pens and checking the condition of birds. However, it was a completely unregulated industry, and no one seemed willing to assume responsibility. Meyer scented an opportunity. When the botulism scare had hit the sales of Californian sardines and other canned foods in the 1920s, the canners had hired Meyer to advise on heat sterilization, establishing safety procedures that soon became standard across America. Now, he proposed a similar technological solution for Californian bird breeders.

His opening came in March 1932 when 125 leading breeders were summoned to a meeting at the Associated Realty Building in Los Angeles. Opening the proceedings, Dr. Giles Porter, the director of the State Department of Public Health with whom Meyer had previously collaborated during the pneumonic plague outbreak in Los Angeles, introduced Meyer as a world authority on psittacosis and someone who could "prove to you, that this is not just a 'scare' but . . . a really serious matter." Meyer began with a review of medical knowledge of psittacosis prior to 1930, then presented the evidence obtained during the pandemic that psittacosis was a filterable virus. "Probably there is a lot of 'hokus-pokus' talk about psittacosis that is not true," he told breeders, but there was no doubt that it was a "highly contagious infection" that could be spread aerially from bird to man via droppings or mucal discharges. This had been proven by the "sad experience" at the Hygienic Laboratory, where nine people had contracted psittacosis merely after passing along a corridor close to cages containing desiccated material. "Probably the wind blew the dust from these cages through a crack in the door and in this way the contact was made," he said. Next, he briefly detailed his own investigations in San Francisco. Then, pointing to a chart, he directly addressed the problem of infections in bird breeding establishments.

> Let us say, for the sake of argument, we have one hundred birds. In this group of one hundred birds, the disease, parrot fever, breaks out. Probably—let us say—ten of the birds will die. Now these ten birds should have been examined. Unfortunately, nothing of this sort is usually done, but so far, we examine these birds and find ten have the parrot fever. There are ninety birds left. You would probably assume that these ninety birds . . . are practically safe. My answer is NO! NO!

The difficulty was that every pen contained a certain percentage of "carriers"; that is, birds whose spleens showed evidence of prior infection but who did not appear sick or visibly diseased. These healthy-looking birds might harbor the virus for six months or longer without infecting other birds in the same pen. However, if such birds were exposed to cold or sudden climatic changes, then these infections could "become activated," and the birds might "secrete the virus," infecting other birds with whom they were confined. In particular, Meyer speculated, there was a good chance they would pass the virus to young birds or "runts." Nor was that the end of the danger. "Convalescent birds," that is birds recovering from infection, might also secrete the virus for between four to six weeks. In all probability, the only birds that were safe were those with inherited immunity, or older birds that had acquired immunity during previous outbreaks or through exposure to the virus in the nest.

The only way to know for sure whether a flock was infected or not was for breeders to turn over 10 to 20 percent of their stock so that

Meyer could examine them for latent infections. In this way, Meyer would be able to give those aviaries that were free of disease a clean bill of health, and there would be no need for further embargos or quarantines. However, Meyer warned, autopsying the birds was dangerous and expensive work, and, in return, he would expect breeders to pay him for his services. $10,000 should be sufficient.

> This is a disease which has caused in every laboratory they work
> with cases of psittacosis; and we have to almost put our foot in
> the grave, so to speak, in order to solve the problem. I took this
> responsibility to work with you. I therefore solicit from you your
> earnest cooperation—or, I give it up. It is not my business to die
> for a disease like psittacosis.

Not surprisingly, the breeders balked at Meyer's offer, feeling his price was too steep. Instead, they tried to convince health officials that such tests were unnecessary and that once birds reached the age of four months they no longer presented a health risk. Next, they proposed that officials introduce a permit system. Porter refused to budge, but the breeders lobbied the governor, who relented and lifted the embargo. As the trade resumed in the summer of 1931 and parakeets were sent from California to markets in the East, Meyer feared a revival of the pandemic. Once the parakeets reached dealers in New York, there was no telling how many flocks might be infected or in which state or country a psittacosis carrier might turn up next. By the end of the year, Californian lovebirds had been scattered to every state in the union. They proved particularly popular at country fairs in Wisconsin and Minnesota, where they were raffled as prizes. Then, on September 22, 1932, came the news that Mrs. William E. Borah, the wife of the senator from Idaho, was seriously ill at her home in Boise, Idaho. On investigation, her physician discovered she was a collector of parakeets and had recently acquired a set of lovebirds from California. Suspecting parrot fever, her husband, the senator, wired Washington to send serum immediately. Thus began another extraordinary chapter in the history of the Hygienic.

≪≫

TWO MONTHS AFTER McCoy's fumigation of the north building, Congress had passed an act changing the laboratory's name to the National Institute of Health (NIH) and establishing fellowships for research into basic biological and medical problems. The Randsell Act, named after Senator E. Randsell, a Democrat from Louisiana, was seen as a reward for the PHS's investigations of psittacosis and the heroism of its research staff, and marked a sea change in American attitudes to the public funding of medical research.* Unfortunately, when Senator Borah's request arrived on McCoy's desk, the NIH's stores of serum had been exhausted. It was at this point that Armstrong volunteered his services. Having made a full recovery, it was likely his blood still contained antibodies. Why not make use of it? Armstrong's personal physician performed the phlebotomy, then stayed up all night separating out the serum. Because of the urgency, there was no time to check that it was sterile. Instead, the serum was dispatched directly to a waiting plane. The story of the mercy flight was a media sensation, with the Associated Press and national and local newspapers publishing hourly logs of the serum's progress from Washington to Boise, Idaho. By now Mrs. Borah was close to death and her doctors were doubtful the serum would make a difference. But they decided it was worth a try and administered all twelve ounces (350 ml) in a single transfusion. Five days later she was on the road to recovery and by the following February she was fit enough to

---

* It also appears to have been motivated by the 1928–1929 influenza epidemic, the worst flu outbreak since the 1918 pandemic, and chemists' desire to apply their knowledge to medical problems. In 1948, the institute's name was pluralized to National Institutes of Health.

travel to Washington. Her first stop was the NIH. "I came to thank you for saving my life," she told Armstrong. "I have some of your blood flowing through my veins."

If Mrs. Borah's recovery was good news for the NIH, it was bad news for Californian bird breeders, as no sooner had his wife recovered than Senator Borah urged President Hoover to reinstate the embargo, but this time on Californian rather than Argentine birds. Hoover forwarded the request to PHS, prompting Cumming to issue an order banning the interstate transport of Californian parakeets. However, he indicated that if California could find a procedure for demonstrating that its birds were free of psittacosis then he might make an exception. The previous March, breeders had done everything they could to avoid submitting their birds to testing. Now, as the embargo bit, denying them access to lucrative markets in the East, they came around to Meyer's proposition.

By 1933 Meyer and Eddie had inspected sixty-six aviaries containing nearly 2,000 lovebirds. In these aviaries, they found that anywhere from 10 to 90 percent of birds classed as healthy by their owners might be carrying latent psittacosis. However, they observed that while many of these infections were of an "eminently chronic character," they did not spread to parakeets in adjacent pens. Contrary to breeders' claims that they never fell ill, Meyer and Eddie discovered many had antibodies to psittacosis, suggesting they had been previously exposed and had suffered mild infections which had been misdiagnosed. The principal risk came from handling dead birds or direct contact with their nasal discharges and excreta, or from bite wounds. However, on occasion, psittacosis could be contracted simply by inhaling desiccated droppings. Indeed, Meyer found that such droppings were highly efficient aerosols and could be scattered over a wide area simply by the flapping of a bird's wings when it became agitated. In such circumstances, the environment is "charged with virus and becomes a menace to human beings who inhale it." For this reason, they warned, psittacosis presented a particular threat to bird breeders and pet store owners, or those with close attachments to lovebirds.

They also found that the LCL bodies of psittacosis could be readily observed on a microscopic slide simply by taking a smear from the spleens of diseased birds and adding an appropriate stain. In other cases, the size of the spleen provided a rough-and-ready approximation of the degree of a latent infection in a pen. In particular, medium-sized spleens measuring three to five millimeters were more likely to produce "a typical, acutely fatal, or latent" illness in inoculated mice than spleens measuring seven to ten millimeters. Meyer and Eddie also found proportionately more enlarged spleens (six millimeters or greater) in young, immature birds than in the older capped birds, suggesting that parakeets typically contracted psittacosis early in their development and that enlarged but noninfective spleens in the older caged birds was evidence of an old sterilizing infection. Their conclusion was unequivocal: "In general, 'noncapped' immature birds are more frequently carriers of the virus than the 'capped' old birds." The implications were clear: birds needed to be observed until they were at least four months old to be sure that they had cleared the infection and no longer presented a danger of transmitting the mycobacterium.

By 1934 Meyer and Eddie had tested nearly 30,000 parakeets and certified 185 Californian aviaries as psittacosis-free. The program was a valuable source of income for the Hooper Foundation, and soon Meyer was using the funds to investigate other scientific questions. Meyer was not only a bacteriologist and veterinary pathologist, he also considered himself a biologist and nascent ecologist. Though trained in the German tradition, by the 1930s he was growing disenchanted with bacteriology's narrow focus on microbes. Instead, as he considered the phenomenon of latent infections, he found himself drawn to the language of "hosts" and "parasites" and wider evolutionary questions about the relationship between virulence and immunity to disease. In particular, he wished to discover whether wild parakeets showed the same susceptibility to psittacosis as birds bred in captivity. To find out, Meyer paid a barber on a Pacific liner to bring him two hundred wild shell parakeets from the Australian bush. As psittacosis had never been reported in Australian parakeets before, Meyer assumed that these birds would possess a high susceptibility to the virus and lend themselves to comparative exposure and immunity tests. Imagine his astonishment, then, when within four weeks of his quarantining the Australian parakeets, one of them died. On examination he found its spleen riddled with the same lesions as those in the Californian birds. Perhaps the most significant finding, however, came when Meyer allowed the Australian birds to mingle freely with Californian parakeets, half of whom he knew to be latently infected: none of the Australian parakeets died of the disease, and when he sacrificed the birds and performed autopsies, Meyer was unable to recover virus from the birds' spleens.

In an example of Meyer's use of international scientific networks, he immediately shared his findings with the Australian virus researcher Frank Macfarlane Burnet, prompting Burnet to launch a parallel study in which he found that psittacosis was an endemic infection of wild Australian parakeets and had probably been "enzootic amongst Australian parrots for centuries." Burnet hypothesized that it was most likely Australian parrots and parakeets from Japanese dealers, not Argentine parrots, that had been the source of the outbreaks of psittacosis in California in 1931. In a letter to Meyer, Burnet explained that in the wild, young birds were typically infected in the nest, but these natural, mild infections could also flare up under the stress of close confinement, resulting in the birds' losing their acquired resistance and shedding the virus. By questioning importers, Meyer established it was common practice for shippers to mix wild unbanded birds with clean birds, greatly facilitating the spread of the virus. He concluded that in the wild, these virus strains were highly adapted to their avian hosts, but conditions in shipping containers and Californian aviaries had greatly increased the virulence of psittacosis and, as he put it, "shifted the balance in favor of the virus"—hence the spillovers of enzootic psittacosis infections seen in Californian birds and people in the early 1930s.

TODAY, PSITTACOSIS no longer presents a pressing health threat and parrot fever has once again disappeared from public view. The disease's retreat from popular consciousness is due in large part to Meyer. Following the discovery of Aureomycin in 1948, Meyer approached the Hartz Mountain Distribution Company, then the largest supplier of milled bird seed in the United States, to develop a line of medicated millet. By the middle 1950s another easy-to-administer antibiotic, oral tetracycline, had also become available and chlortetracycline-impregnated seed had become standard in the bird breeding industry. To be sure, there were still occasional outbreaks, but these tended to occur on turkey farms or in poultry processing plants, where exposure to psittacosis was, and still is, an occupational hazard. In most cases, all it took was a properly administered course of tetracycline to clear human infections and return a flock to health.

Unfortunately, today, as in the 1930s, some breeders refuse to believe their aviaries are latently infected. Instead, they dilute the seed or fail to administer a full course of antibiotics, resulting in the persistence of subclinical infections of psittacosis in domestic bird flocks. Should these birds be shipped to a pet store and mingle with imported birds emerging from quarantine, there is a risk they will communicate the organism and spark fresh outbreaks of parrot fever. Indeed, the principal lesson of the 1930 pandemic is that imported birds were merely the fall guys. The main culprits were domestic lovebirds bred in Californian aviaries. Once this was realized, parrots and parakeets ceased to be a source of fear and hysteria, and the control of psittacosis

became a largely veterinary problem. However, without the simultaneous worldwide outbreaks sparked by Argentinian parrots and the
press coverage that accompanied it, it is unlikely that anyone would
have noticed the unusual pattern of pneumonia deaths, and Nocard's
error that psittacosis was due to a type of salmonella would have taken
longer to dispel.

There was another lesson, too, one that would become increasingly
apposite in the second half of the twentieth century as other little-
known or neglected pathogens emerged to spark new epidemic scares.
And that is that in nature parrots and parakeets pose little threat to
human populations. Sure, there might be occasional mass die-offs
deep in the Amazonian rain forest or the Australian bush, but, in
Burnet's words, psittacosis was "not intrinsically a very infectious disease." On the contrary, he argued, the parasite's primary function was
to return wild bird populations that had grown too large or too dense
for their ecological niches to a state of equilibrium. The problem was
that when man disrupted these biological and ecological processes by
packing parakeets into overcrowded crates, he created the ideal conditions for the propagation of the virus and its transfer from bird to
man. "It is reasonably certain that cockatoos, left to a natural life in
the wild, would never have shown any symptoms of their infection,"
Burnet observed, following an outbreak in Melbourne in 1935. "In
captivity, crowded, filthy and without exercise or sunlight, a flare-up
of any latent infection was only to be expected."

Indeed, by the 1940s Burnet was worrying that these spillover
events were becoming more common and that overpopulation, coupled with international trade and jet travel, was disrupting natural
ecologies in new and unpredictable ways, leading to virulent outbreaks
of vector-borne diseases such as yellow fever. While a world in which
everyone and everything was more closely linked in a biological sense
should favor a "virtual equilibrium" between humans and microbial

parasites, Burnet warned that "man . . . lives in an environment constantly being changed by his own activities, and few of his diseases have attained such equilibrium."

Meyer also worried about the way that rapid economic and industrial change was disrupting the balance between humans and microbes. However, in the case of psittacosis he placed the blame squarely on bird breeders and their stubborn insistence that psittacosis did not pose a threat, even as the disease claimed the lives of pet owners and medical researchers in Baltimore and Washington. Perhaps the most important factor of all, however, had been the popularity of lovebirds with American consumers and the lucrative interstate trade that saw itinerant peddlers going door-to-door offering parakeets to widows and housewives. In 1930, the idea that these cute American-bred birds might be the avian equivalent of Trojan horses was too disturbing to contemplate. Far easier to blame feathered green immigrants from the southern hemisphere.

CHAPTER IV

THE "PHILLY KILLER"

"The outbreak . . . has presented a number of unusual and
complex features. . . . It has run counter to our expectations
that contemporary science is infallible and can solve all
the problems that we confront."
—DAVID J. SENCER, director, CDC,
Atlanta, November 24, 1976

At the junction of Walnut Street and South Broad Street—or what Philadelphians now call the "Avenue of the Arts"— stands a well-appointed modern business hotel. With its spacious guestrooms boasting "pillow top" mattresses and its wood-paneled nineteenth-floor restaurant with sweeping views over Center City, the Hyatt at the Bellevue effortlessly combines contemporary luxury and old-world charm. That charm is evident the moment you step from Broad Street into the lobby area and glide across the polished floor to the reception desk, taking in the glittering chandelier overhead and the curved staircase with its elegant hand-worked marble-and-iron rails. However, if you care little for decor and have important business to attend to, the hotel also offers state-of-the-art conference rooms, plus an indoor jogging track, a full-length swimming pool, and a 93,000-square-foot sports club. For allergy sufferers or the hyper-health-conscious, the Hyatt at the Bellevue even has spotless "hypo-allergenic" rooms equipped with a high-tech air purification system designed to filter out allergens and other airborne irritants.

"Enjoy a better night's sleep and make the most of your travels in a Hyatt PURE room," reads the hotel's marketing blurb.

What is not mentioned anywhere on the hotel's website is the thing the building is best known for, at least among members of Philadelphia's baby boom generation. For in 1976, the Bellevue-Stratford, as the hotel was then known, was the site of one of the most baffling infectious disease outbreaks in history—an outbreak centered on the hotel's air conditioning and water cooling systems.

The "Legionnaires' disease" affair began on Wednesday, July 21, when 2,300 delegates from the Pennsylvania section of the American Legion and their families (some 4,500 people in all) began arriving at the Bellevue-Stratford for their annual four-day jamboree. It was the summer of the American Bicentennial celebrations, and the Legionnaires—many of them veterans of World War II and Korea—were looking forward to partying in style. Those who could afford it—perhaps five hundred in all—had checked into the Bellevue, taking advantage of the discounts on rooms negotiated by the Legion's state adjutant, Edward Hoak, whose job it was to preside over the convention that year and glad-hand delegates.

Formed from the shell of the Stratford, which used to stand at the southwest corner of Stratford and Broad, and the Bellevue, which used to overlook the northwest corner, the Bellevue-Stratford had opened its doors to guests in 1904 after a two-year refit costing a staggering $8 million (about $20 million in today's money). Billed at the time as the most luxurious hotel in the nation, it was designed in the French Renaissance style, with the most magnificent ballroom in the United States, four restaurants, 1,000 guest rooms, and lighting fixtures by Thomas Edison. By the 1920s, "the Grande Old Dame of Broad Street" had become a fixture of Philadelphia society and a favorite haunt of celebrities, royalty, and heads of state. Former guests included Mark Twain, Rudyard Kipling, Queen Marie of Romania, and General John J. Pershing. Every US president from Theodore Roosevelt on had stayed there, including President John F. Kennedy, who had visited the hotel in October 1963, the month before his assassination in Dallas. However, by the 1970s the Bellevue had fallen out of fashion and was struggling to compete with the new luxury chains. Indeed, despite the discounts negotiated by Hoak, many delegates complained that the food and drinks were overpriced. They also thought the air conditioning in the hospitality suites was substandard and did not like the attitude of the "snooty" staff.

Those who could not afford the Bellevue had opted for the nearby Ben Franklin hotel and other cheaper midtown options. However, nearly everyone had visited the Bellevue's lobby to register and as all the principal conference events, from the Keystone Go-Getter Club Breakfast on the opening day, to the Commander's Bicentennial Ball on the final evening, were held at the hotel, conventioneers and their families soon became familiar with its bars and hospitality suites. The Legionnaires loved a drink at the best of times, and with temperatures in Philadelphia that week in the high nineties, the suites were soon packed with delegates seeking to quench their thirst and cool off. To keep costs down, Hoak had arranged for delegates to supply their own alcohol and snacks, but he could do little about the hotel's creaking air conditioning system or the ice supplies, which soon ran out.

The first intimation Hoak had that Legionnaires had been visited by something worse than a hangover came a week later when he arrived in Manor, Pennsylvania, a small town two hundred miles west of Harrisburg, for the swearing-in of new officers of Post 472 and was informed that six Legionnaires in the area were ill and that one had died. There was further grim news when Hoak returned to his home near Harrisburg and found a letter waiting for him from the wife of a close colleague informing him that her husband was ill with pneumonia and was not responding to treatment. A few hours later Hoak received word from his secretary that the man was dead. Next, Hoak called his assistant adjutant in Chambersburg concerning another matter only to learn that he was attending the viewing of Charles Chamberlain, commander-elect of St. Thomas Post 612 in south-central Pennsylvania, who had died suddenly following the convention. When Hoak called the former state commander of Williamsport to inform him of the three deaths, he learned that six other people from Williamsport who had also attended the convention were seriously ill in area hospitals. In theory this was not unusual. After all, the Legionnaires formed an elderly demographic and many were also heavy smokers and drinkers with underlying health problems. But two deaths and more than six hospitalizations in the space of a week struck Hoak as more than a little odd, and when he made further calls and learned that other delegates across the state were also ill, his alarm deepened.

Hoak was not the only person becoming concerned that weekend. On Saturday, July 31, Robert Sharrar, chief of Acute Communicable Disease Control for Philadelphia, had taken a call from a physician in Carlisle worried about a patient who had recently attended the Legion convention and who was complaining of a fever and a dry, hacking cough. A chest X-ray indicated the patient had bronchopneumonia of the lower right lobe. Sharrar told him it sounded like mycoplasmal pneumonia and advised him to draw blood and send it for testing to the state laboratory when it reopened on Monday. In the meantime, he recommended the doctor treat his patient with a fast-acting antibiotic. Sharrar was about to end the conversation when the doctor asked whether he knew of any other cases of pneumonia in Philadelphia in the past few days. Sharrar did not. That was when the doctor said that he had heard that a patient had recently died of pneumonia in Lewisburg, in northwest Pennsylvania. Sharrar immediately called Lewisburg Hospital and asked to be put through to the resident pathologist, who informed him that the victim was a Legionnaire and that the cause of death had been "acute viral . . . hemorrhagic pneumonia."

Two cases of pneumonia in a city the size of Philadelphia was not unusual—in an average summer week Sharrar could expect twenty to thirty deaths from the disease. Nevertheless, the cases gave Sharrar pause for thought. In February, a new strain of swine flu had been isolated at a US Army base at Fort Dix, New Jersey, thirty-five miles northeast of Philadelphia. The flu had claimed the life of a young private and gone on to sicken several soldiers on the base. Tests showed the strain was closely related to the H1N1 virus responsible for the deadly "Spanish flu" pandemic. Fearing that the Fort Dix outbreak was the harbinger of a new pandemic wave, David Sencer, the director of the CDC in Atlanta, had urged the Ford administration to immunize the entire US population. As a CDC-trained epidemiologist, Sharrar had fully supported Sencer's recommendation and was determined that Philadelphians would be among the first to get the flu shots. All he was waiting for was for Congress to approve the administration's $134 million funding request and for politicians in Washington to agree to insurance to cover vaccine manufacturers worried about their liability should the vaccine prove to have adverse effects.

IN THE LATE VICTORIAN and Edwardian periods, pneumonia had been the most feared disease after tuberculosis and was nearly always fatal, particularly in the case of the elderly or those with compromised immune systems. Indeed, prior to antibiotics, lobar pneumonia had accounted for roughly one-quarter of all deaths in the United States.

However, this changed with Dubos's discovery in 1927, in Avery's laboratory at the Rockefeller Institute in New York, of an enzyme that decomposed the polysaccharide capsule of the pneumococcus, making it vulnerable to phagocytosis. Together with the isolation of the first sulfa drugs in the 1930s, treatment and survival rates for pneumonia gradually improved. The wider availability of penicillin in the late 1940s, and the discovery of new antibiotics such as erythromycin and doxycycline in the 1950s, coupled with better respiratory tech-

nology in hospitals, saw further strides in treatment and convalescent care. By the early 1970s the rate of hospital fatalities had fallen to
around 5 percent, the level at which it remains today. The result was
that pneumonia ceased to be an interesting field of research for young
medical scientists. Instead, believing that the "conquest of epidemic
disease" was imminent, researchers focused on cancer and chronic
diseases associated with genetic conditions and modern lifestyles.

As the outbreak in Philadelphia would demonstrate, this was a mistake. While most bacterial pneumonias are due to the pneumococcus,
pneumonia can also be caused by several other common bacteria, for
example, *Yersinia pestis*, the bacterium of plague, and *Chlamydia psittaci*, the bacterium of psittacosis. Another common source of atypical pneumonias is *Hemophilus influenzae*, the bacillus that Pfeiffer
blamed for the Russian and Spanish influenza pandemics, and *Myco-
plasma pneumoniae*, a tiny organism midway between a bacterium and
a virus. In addition, there had been several outbreaks of pneumonia
for which a causal agent had never been identified. These unsolved
outbreaks included an incident in 1965 at St. Elizabeths Mental Hospital in Washington, DC in which fourteen people had died, and
an outbreak at a health department building in Pontiac, Michigan.
Dubbed "Pontiac Fever," the latter had caused an influenza-like illness in 144 workers and visitors to the building, including a team
from the CDC. Although there had been no deaths and no recorded
cases of pneumonia, guinea pigs exposed to aerosols of unfiltered
water from the building's air condenser unit developed nodular pneumonia. That suggested the presence of a bacterium-sized infectious
agent. Unfortunately, all attempts to culture the pathogen from the
water or from the lung tissue of guinea pigs failed, much to the CDC's
frustration. The result was that while the Pontiac and St. Elizabeths
outbreaks were known to epidemiologists, the cases had never been
written up. By contrast, everyone knew about the swine flu outbreak at
Fort Dix because there was such a panic about it and the newspapers

were full of the government's vaccination plans. Perhaps that was why, on August 2, a physician from the Veterans Administration Clinic in Philadelphia telephoned CDC headquarters and asked to speak with someone from the National Influenza Immunization Program. He was put through to Robert Craven, a young Epidemic Intelligence Service (EIS) officer who, together with his colleague, Phil Graitcer, was manning the desk in Auditorium A, the "war room" set up by the CDC in expectation of a nationwide epidemic of swine flu. The physician had grim news: four Legionnaires admitted to his clinic had died of pneumonia over the weekend. All of them had attended the state convention in Philadelphia. In addition, some twenty-six other people who had been at the convention were also showing signs of "febrile respiratory disease."

At first Craven and Graitcer dismissed the reports: four deaths from pneumonia was to be expected among such a large gathering of elderly people. However, within the hour the CDC officers had fielded several more calls from doctors and health officials in Pennsylvania telling a similar story, and by mid-morning the death count from pneumonia had reached eleven. Now that *was* unusual. As it happened, one of their colleagues, another young EIS officer named Jim Beecham, had recently been posted to the headquarters of the Pennsylvania State Health Department in Harrisburg. When Craven got through to him he learned that earlier that morning Hoak had issued a statement saying that at least eight of his members were dead and some thirty other Legionnaires who had attended the convention were ill with "mysterious symptoms." Reporters wondered whether the cases were connected to swine flu.

Influenza typically has an incubation period of one to four days, and most healthy adults are able to infect others up to five to seven days after becoming sick. If the Legionnaires had caught swine flu at the convention in Philadelphia, then the first illnesses would have shown themselves around July 28. It also meant that officials could expect a second wave in the first week of August. Was that what was now happening? Had the long-feared swine flu outbreak begun? No one was sure, but with rumors mounting and pharmaceutical companies months away from being able to supply sufficient doses of vaccine, it was imperative that the CDC answer the question quickly. If nothing else, David Sencer's reputation depended on it.

The person to whom it fell to investigate the outbreak was David Fraser, a 32-year-old graduate of Harvard Medical School who bore a striking resemblance to Bobby Kennedy. Tapped as a future director of the CDC, Fraser had recently been appointed head of the CDC's Special Pathogens Branch and occupied a small windowless office five floors above the swine flu war room. There he presided over a crack team of epidemiologists, including the latest cohort of EIS graduates. Established in 1951 as an early warning corps against biological warfare, EIS is the CDC's elite disease detection squad. As befits a group that takes pride in its ability to investigate outbreaks in any part of the world, its symbol is a globe with a worn-out shoe sole. Every year, between 250 to 300 applicants compete for the privilege of seventy-five places in the EIS's intensive, two-year training program. Candidates are recruited from every area of medicine and include doctors, veterinarians, virologists, nurses, and dentists. The emphasis is on applied epidemiological procedures, biostatistics, and the management of an outbreak investigation. Particular emphasis is placed on the study of old case files and the compilation of "line lists," or charts, detailing each case and the distribution of infections in time and space. In addition, trainees are expected to learn how to gather pathology and serology specimens.

In keeping with the vision of EIS's founder, Alexander D. Langmuir, the emphasis was on learning on the job. As Langmuir once told an interviewer, he liked nothing better than throwing EIS candidates "overboard" to see if they could swim; and if they couldn't, he was happy to "throw them a life ring, pull them out, and throw them in again." In short, EIS graduates would stop at nothing to get to the bottom of an outbreak. A few years earlier, for instance, Fraser had helped solve the mystery of a Lassa Fever outbreak in Sierra Leone that had very nearly killed one of his colleagues who tramped through villages trapping rodents in search of the presumed reservoir of the virus (he eventually traced it to a local species of brown rat). Another reason Sencer had picked Fraser was his reputation for diplomacy, something that Sencer knew would be needed when Fraser arrived in Harrisburg, the Pennsylvania state capital, and local health officials learned of the CDC's interest in the case.

The first thing epidemiologists are taught in the event of an outbreak is to draw up a working case definition in order to verify the diagnosis. The second is to look at the frequency of exposure among people with illness and those of comparable groups who are not ill (so-called controls). Only then is it possible to say whether the identified cases constitute an epidemic. As Fraser left for Harrisburg on August 3, he knew there were one hundred suspected cases and that there had been nineteen deaths. He also knew that all the cases involved Legionnaires who had attended the state convention in Philadelphia. However, that could merely be an artifact of the reporting: the American Legion was a close-knit group with efficient communication networks, so it was only natural that cases occurring among Legionnaires would come to attention first. Moreover, the press was already showing a keen interest in the outbreak, something that was likely to further skew the reporting. To know if there really was an epidemic underway in Pennsylvania, Fraser would need to establish whether any other groups or individuals had also fallen ill with pneumonia in the relevant time period and whether they had also been in Philadelphia or somewhere else. He would also need to establish how many Legionnaires and their families had attended the convention so as to obtain an accurate denominator with which to gauge the attack rate. Ideally, he would also need line lists detailing the name, age, and address of each patient, and, in the case of Legionnaires, the dates they had attended the convention and the hotels they had stayed at. These charts would also need to include key medical and pathological information, such as the date of onset of illness and, in the case of the deceased, the cause of death. Clearly it was a big job, and before it had ended thirty EIS officers had fanned out across the state, interviewing the families of victims or, in the case of those who had been hospitalized, the institutions where they had received treatment. In anticipation of this effort, on August 2 the CDC had dispatched Craven and Graitcer to Pittsburgh and Philadelphia respectively, and a recently qualified EIS officer, Theodore Tsai, to Harrisburg. In addition, Fraser would be joined in Harrisburg by two other newly qualified EIS officers, David Heymann, a future director of Emerging and Communicable Diseases at the World Health Organization, and Stephen Thacker, who would go on to become an assistant surgeon general in the US Public Health Service.

The other priority was to establish whether or not the outbreak was due to swine flu. This task would largely fall to Graitcer, whose job it was to liaise with state laboratories and forward throat washings and sera to the CDC's laboratory in Atlanta. There, a team of specialists was on hand to see if the sera cross-reacted with the H1N1 swine flu, dubbed A/New Jersey/76, that had been isolated at Fort Dix in February. At the same time, CDC technicians would test for antigens to the most prevalent strain of flu then circulating in the northern hemisphere, an H3N2 virus known as A/Victoria/75, as well as other common infectious agents associated with pneumonia.

Within forty-eight hours of arriving in Harrisburg, Fraser had the answer to the first question: it was not swine flu. And within seventy-two hours technicians confirmed it was not the A/New Jersey or A/Victoria strains either. That left several other possibilities. At the top of the list was *Chlamydia psittaci*, the bacterium of psittacosis, and *Coxiella burnetii*, the bacterium of Q fever, a disease of cattle, sheep, and goats which was also known to cause pneumonia in humans. Another more remote possibility was *Histoplasma*, a fungal infection transmitted by birds and bats. Testing for these pathogens, Fraser knew, would take weeks and possibly months, and would have to be combined with the calm and careful collection of other evidence, such as dust and water samples from the Bellevue, and the examination of pathology specimens from deceased Legionnaires. But arriving at the offices of Leonard Bachmann, the secretary of health for Pennsylvania, and his chief epidemiologist, William Parkin, Fraser found the atmosphere anything but calm. Already, the phones were ringing off the hook with panicked callers, while in the press room next door newspapermen were demanding to know whether the outbreak might be something more sinister, a deliberate act of poisoning perhaps done by antiwar radicals intent on sabotaging the Bicentennial celebrations or sending a message to Gerald Ford, who two years earlier had controversially pardoned Richard Nixon for his alleged crimes in connection with the Watergate break-in. The press could be forgiven for asking such questions; in the run-up to the convention, Philadelphia's mayor, Frank Rizzo, a tough-talking former policeman and close friend of Nixon's, had deliberately stoked fears of a terrorist attack by posting undercover officers in and around the downtown area. Following the outbreak, Rizzo's official spokesman, Albert Gaudiosi, had raised even more bizarre conspiracy theories, including the possibility of a covert operation by the CIA using chemical and biological weapons. Gaudiosi's statement struck many as a blatant attempt to divert attention from the mayor's failure to resolve a long-running garbage collection dispute—a dispute that had gone on for three weeks and had seen mounds of refuse collect on city streets. Those garbage mounds were a magnet for rats and other vermin. Might those rats be infested with plague fleas? wondered journalists. Could plague be the source of the Legionnaires' peculiar pneumonic symptoms?

While CDC scientists were testing sputa and examining lung tissue and other pathology specimens, EIS officers were extending their investigations across Pennsylvania. Each officer drove an average of 450 miles, interviewing ten patients in over six hospitals. By now, a clear clinical picture was emerging. Typically, a case of Legionnaires' disease began with a feeling of malaise, muscle aches, and a slight headache. Within twenty-four hours, patients would exhibit a rapidly rising fever, chills, and a dry cough, as well as, on occasion, abdominal pains and gastrointestinal symptoms. Two or three days later, the patients would have a raging fever of 102–105°F, and a chest X-ray would show patchy pneumonia. Accordingly, a case was defined clinically as any person with a cough or fever of 102°F or higher, or any fever and chest X-ray evidence of pneumonia. In addition, investigators included an epidemiological criterion (a case must have attended the American Legion convention or been inside the Bellevue-Stratford between July 1 and August 18). At this point, the cases listed at the State Department of Health consisted entirely of people who had attended the convention or who had been at the Bellevue, so this clinico-epidemiological definition made sense. However, it was also possible that the line lists had been skewed by the publicity surrounding the outbreak at the Bellevue and that people had not thought to report other cases that might warrant inclusion, so the Department of Health also set up a hotline and invited members of the public to report possible epidemic cases regardless of association with the convention or the Bellevue.

By the first week of August it was clear that the epidemic had peaked and the disease was not contagious, there being no secondary cases. Tracing the epidemic curve back in time, it was evident there had been a rapid upswing in cases from July 22 to 25, followed by a plateau through July 28 and a somewhat slow decline through August 3. Moreover, there had been no cases prior to the convention, suggesting that, whatever the agent, the incubation period was two to ten days. In all, in a four-week period up to August 10, there had been

182 cases and 29 deaths, giving a case fatality rate of 16 percent. The infection had proved particularly dangerous to cigarette smokers and older age groups, with those aged sixty or more twice as likely to suffer fatal outcomes. Almost all were Legionnaires who had either resided at the Bellevue or had attended events in its lobby and hospitality suites. However, there were also a few clinically compatible cases among non-Legionnaires. These included a Bellevue air conditioner repair man, a bus driver, and several pedestrians who had merely passed by the hotel's imposing frontage on Broad Street. Were these Broad Street pneumonias part of the same epidemiological event? And why was it that, with the exception of the air conditioner repair man, hardly any of the Bellevue's employees appeared to have fallen ill?

Though epidemiology aspires to be an exact science, it also contains a large element of induction. As Wade Hampton Frost, a former professor of epidemiology at Johns Hopkins and one of the pioneers of the field, once put it: "Epidemiology at any given time is something more than the total of its established facts. It includes their orderly arrangement into chains of inference which extend beyond the bounds of direct observation." In other words, the raw data can only be parsed so far. To get a feel for Legionnaires' disease, Fraser realized he needed to go to the focus of the outbreak. Obtaining rooms at the Bellevue was not a problem: by now, most guests had canceled their bookings for fear of contracting the disease, and on August 10 Fraser and ten of his officers moved into the hotel and began exploring the lobby area and hospitality suites. Was there a pattern, he wondered, some sort of clue in the way that the Legionnaires had used the hotel's facilities?

To verify how many of the 10,000 registered Pennsylvania Legion members had actually attended the convention and to reconstruct their movements, Fraser distributed questionnaires to Legionnaires across the state. As well as confirming their attendance in Philadelphia, Legionnaires were asked to provide details of which hotel they had stayed at, and how many hours they had spent inside the Bellevue or on the sidewalk outside. The two-page questionnaires also contained checklists about key convention activities and functions. Had they gone to the Keystone Go-Getter Club Breakfast on the morning of July 23 in the Rose Garden on the eighteenth floor of the Bellevue? Had they attended the ticket-only Commander's Bicentennial Ball in the Bellevue's lavish second floor ballroom that same evening? Fraser also quizzed them about their consumption of food, coffee, and alcohol, and whether they had added ice and mixers to their drinks or bought anything from street vendors during the Legion parade through downtown. In addition, officers interviewed other guests and nonconventioneers who had stayed at or visited the Bellevue during the same period. Finally, EIS officers interviewed Bellevue staff to establish whether they had suffered any illnesses. To help with the surveys, Rizzo even provided Fraser and Sharrar with a team of homicide detectives. According to Sharrar, the detectives "did not miss a trick" and proved particularly adept at quizzing Legionnaires about their interactions with female sex workers, many of whom had passed themselves off as hotel guests in order to gain access to the hospitality suites.

It quickly became apparent that nearly everyone had spent time in the first floor lobby area, where the registration desk was set up, talking to other delegates running for election or chatting to family and friends. And nearly everyone had ridden in the elevators, either to visit the rooftop restaurant or to visit the bars and hospitality suites. Typical cases included Jimmy Dolan and John Bryant Ralph—"J.D" and "J.B." in the anonymous line lists. Members of the Williamstown Legion post, Dolan and Ralph were thirty-nine and forty-one respectively and had been buddies since childhood. To save money, the pair had stayed at the Holiday Inn in midtown with Jimmy's cousin, Richard Dolan, the forty-three-year-old commander of Pennsylvania Legion Post 239. Well built and with a reputation for partying, all three had attended the Commander's Bicentennial ball, drinking until well past midnight. The trio had also spent many hours in the lobby area, but had avoided the hotel's bars and restaurants. Within days of returning to Williamstown, both Jimmy Dolan and Ralph were complaining of fever, headaches, and coughs, and on July 29 Jimmy Dolan was admitted to the hospital. He died three days later, the pathologist recording the cause as "bilateral consolidation lungs, bloody sputum terminal." The day after, August 2, Ralph also succumbed to the mysterious disease, the cause of death being listed as "gross massive bilateral lobar pneumonia." By contrast, Richard Dolan had suffered no symptoms of illness.

Three "statistically significant" factors emerged from the questionnaires. First, ill delegates had spent on average four or five more hours in the Bellevue than had healthy delegates, and considerably more time in the lobby than controls. The correlation between the amount of time spent in the lobby and illness applied particularly to those who had slept at the Bellevue, but also held for Legionnaires who had stayed at other hotels. However, this correlation did not hold for hotel staff who worked in the lobby area and had spent as much if not more time there than Legionnaires. Indeed, with the exception of an air conditioning repair man, who had developed flu-like symptoms on July 21 and had returned to work four days later, there was no evidence of illness or disease in any of the hotel's thirty full-time employees. Second, there appeared to be a small correlation between illness and visits to hospitality suites, with delegate cases visiting on average 2.6 hospitality rooms as compared to 1.8 visited by nondelegate cases. However, no one hospitality room had been visited by more than one-third of cases. Third, while cases were more likely to have drunk water at the Bellevue than noncases, only two-thirds admitted to drinking water in any form, presumably because they preferred to quench their thirst with alcohol and/or carbonated drinks. In short, as Sharrar put it, the typical case "was most likely to be a friendly, thirsty, elderly, male delegate who hung around the hotel lobby."

In any outbreak investigation, once the existence of the epidemic has been confirmed and the diagnosis established, the next questions are who, where, when, how, and what? Following the surveys, there could be little doubt that Legionnaires were the who, the convention was the when, and the Bellevue was the where. But that left the how and what wide open. Had Legionnaires' disease been triggered by exposure to a fomite, such as dust or ash particles, or was it due to some kind of gas? Alternatively, could the pathogen have been water- or food-borne? Moreover, if the common denominator was the Bellevue, how did one explain the apparent immunity of the hotel's staff? Was it possible that the conspiracy theories were right and the outbreak had been a deliberate act of espionage?

By now, speculation was rife, with several newspapers suggesting the Legionnaires had been poisoned with paraquat, a weed killer known to cause pulmonary edema and breathing problems. Another suggestion was phosgene gas, a pulmonary agent that had been deployed by the Germans, and later the Allies, in World War I, which causes choking and shortness of breath. Other suggestions were that the Legionnaires' symptoms could be due to poisoning with nickel carbonyl, a highly toxic liquid that can trigger chemical pneumonitis and cardiorespiratory failure, or else cadmium poisoning from the cadmium pitchers that the bar staff had used to mix the Legionnaires' drinks. Fraser asked CDC technicians to screen pathology specimens from the deceased Legionnaires for traces of these toxins and poisons and instructed EIS officers to examine the restaurants, bars, rooms, and hospitality suites for traces of the same chemicals. If the pathogen had been phosgene, Fraser reasoned, it could have been added to the Legionnaires' drinks or sucked in gaseous form via the elevator shaft, from where the constant motion of the elevators would have distributed it to the upper floors of the hotel. That could be why the survey had turned up no association between the illness and Legionnaires' presence in a particular hospitality suite. However, everyone had ridden the elevators and had gotten in and out at the lobby. Phosgene is also rapidly excreted from the body, making it an ideal poisoning agent. However, it usually causes severe kidney damage, and none of the kidneys from Legionnaires exhibited signs of trauma. Nor did any of the specimens contain paraquat. By contrast, traces of nickel were found in the lungs, liver, and kidneys of six Legionnaires and two of the Broad Street pneumonias. However, these were well within normal levels and were not elevated compared to those of controls.

As the obvious candidates were excluded, Fraser began to consider more remote possibilities, including the air conditioning system. Most modern hotels boast rooftop chiller units, as cold air settles and it is impossible to drive cold air upwards. However, the Bellevue employed an old cold water system operated via two Carrier refrigeration machines located in the subbasement. Installed in 1954, these chillers had a capacity of 800 and 600 tons respectively and used Freon 11 refrigerant to cool the water. This chilled water was then pumped up to the roof of the hotel from where it was circulated downward to some sixty air-handling units (AHUs). Most of these used approximately 75 percent recirculated air and 25 percent outside air, but in the case of the AHU located directly above the lobby desk, all of the air was recirculated.

At the same time, a separate system, using "cooled" water from a cooling tower on the roof, was employed to condense the refrigerant. In the event of accidental leakage, the chilled water system was designed to be replenished automatically via a float valve in a nearby water expansion tank. Unfortunately, due to a fault in the valve, the water pipes at the top of the hotel had become filled with air, resulting in the failure of one of the AHUs serving the Rose Garden restaurant on the eighteenth floor. To rectify this, staff had hooked up a temporary connection using a garden hose that ran from the water tower to a pipe leading to the AHU. This makeshift system solved the problem of the faulty float in the expansion tank, but if the valves at either end

of the hose were left open or leaked and various safety valves malfunc-
tioned, it was conceivable that water from the water tower could have
found its way into two steel tanks, also located in the roof, that supplied the hotel's drinking water. Since the water in the tower had been
treated with chromate to preserve the pipes, this made it a potential
contamination risk. The water tower was also uncovered and exposed
to the elements, meaning it would be very easy for droppings from
pigeons roosting on the balconies to get into the potable water.

Another potentially worse hazard was the 800-ton basement chiller
unit. The unit had been leaking F-11 coolant continuously since May,
prompting the Bellevue's management to put in repeated calls to
the Carrier company to fix the problem. However, these repairs had
been only partly successful, and with the summer conference season
imminent, management had opted to postpone further servicing until
later in the year. Unfortunately, air from the subbasement exhausted
directly onto Chancellor Street on the southern side of the hotel. In
theory the exhausted air could have contained F-11 coolant from the
faulty chiller in a gaseous state. In addition, piped vents from the chillers also discharged air onto Chancellor Street just three feet away from
the exhaust fan, meaning it was possible that some of this air could
have been sucked back into the subbasement via an air shaft adjacent
to the point of exhaust. Fraser was unable to determine the "ultimate
fate of this air," but as the subbasement was also served by two large
fans that exhausted air via another shaft that extended up to the roof,
he could not discount the possibility that contaminated air had been
circulated throughout the hotel. Fueling Fraser's suspicions about
leaking chiller coolant was the fact that an air conditioner repair man
had signed off sick on July 20, the day before the convention opened.
As the man reported having a cough and a temperature of 102°F, his
name had been included in the line list. However, he did not develop
pneumonia and on July 24 was well enough to return to work. Later,
it was discovered that his wife and two daughters had been sick with a

respiratory illness at the same time, prompting Sharrar to argue that he should never have been included in the line list and that his illness was probably due to flu, not Legionnaires' disease.

By the end of August, EIS officers had combed the hotel from top to bottom. Samples removed to Atlanta for testing included Freon 11 and chilled water from the air conditioner system; dust from the AHUs, carpets, draperies, and hotel elevators; water from the hotel drinking fountains and ice dispensers; rodent control chemicals; bleaches and housekeeping supplies; and a variety of convention mementos including mugs, hats, badges, and packs of Merit cigarettes that had been included in the convention gift bags. Noticing that ventilation grilles from the subway discharged onto Broad Street, Fraser had also ordered inspections of the underground concourse. Finally, mindful that no epidemiological survey could be considered complete without a record of the weather, Fraser ordered up meteorological readings for the period from July 21 to 25. These showed that the convention had opened to sweltering conditions and that on July 22 there had been a sharp temperature inversion. The result was that rather than temperatures decreasing with elevation above ground level, as is usual, air at the upper levels of the hotel, including the roof, had become superheated. This unusual effect had lasted for a day and a half, ending at around noon on July 24, and, Fraser discovered, had been accompanied by slightly higher levels of carbon monoxide and other atmospheric pollutants.

From the beginning, one of the most popular theories was that the outbreak had been due to psittacosis. Although in 1976 the great parrot fever pandemic of 1930 was a distant memory, ornithologists and veterinary specialists had continued to study the epidemiology of the disease and its natural history. As tighter regulation reduced the incidence of outbreaks in bird breeding establishments and pet stores, the focus had shifted to occupational settings, such as turkey farms and poultry processing plants. At the same time, serological studies and a better understanding of the role of latent infections had brought a new appreciation of the disease's wide host range. Indeed, in 1967, Karl Meyer had tabulated 130 species of bird that carried the disease. These included homing pigeons raised in backyard lofts and the pigeons in New York's Central Park, half of whom were found to be harboring the chlamydia bacterium.

Fraser noted that the upper floors and roof of the Bellevue were popular pigeon roosts. In addition, a local Philadelphia character, known as the "pigeon lady," had been seen scattering bread crumbs on Broad Street. Then, there was the report from a guest that she had heard a parakeet chirping in one of the rooms. Fraser's task was not made any easier by the support given to the psittacosis theory by prominent medics. The most vocal was Dr. Gary Lattimer, a specialist in infectious diseases at the Sacred Heart Hospital in Allentown. In early August, Lattimer had examined four Legionnaires and, believing they had psittacosis, treated them with tetracycline, a broad-spectrum antibiotic that was known to be effective against psittacosis and rickettsial diseases.* The Legionnaires' symptoms had immediately improved, prompting Lattimer to urge Fraser to issue a directive recommending tetracycline to other patients. Fraser refused, citing the absence of scientific proof and saying it would be irresponsible to recommend tetracycline over erythromycin and rifampicin. However, Lattimer would not back down. Instead he began holding press conferences and writing to well-known chlamydia experts, including Julius Schachter, Meyer's former pupil and a professor of epidemiology at UCSF. In support of his theory, Lattimer cited the fact that psittacosis had a variable incubation period of three to eleven days, similar to the two to ten days' period for Legionnaires' disease. The mortality rate and symp-

---

* *Rickettsia* is the name for a family of bacteria transmitted by the bites of chiggers, ticks, fleas, and lice. The best known rickettsial diseases are typhus and Rocky Mountain Spotted Fever.

toms were also similar, and, as with psittacosis, there appeared to be no secondary transmission. Finally, Lattimer pointed out that histopathological examinations revealed extensive alveolitis or inflammation of the air sacs of victims' lungs. Together with the changes seen in the liver and spleen, these were "compatible in all aspects with those reported from previous human chlamydial epidemics." Unfortunately for Lattimer, in September a panel of expert pathologists tasked with reviewing the autopsy evidence disagreed. Although the panel found that five of the core Legionnaires cases and the three Broad Street pneumonias showed patterns of "acute diffuse alveolar damage," it ruled that such alveolar damage could also be the result of exposure to toxins. "No pathologic diagnosis could be made on the basis of these findings," they concluded.

All hope of solving the mystery now rested on the microbiology studies. As the leading federal agency for disease control and a WHO reporting center for influenza, the CDC's laboratories in Atlanta were considered second to none. Staffed by 625 scientists and technicians, the laboratories, which were located on the main Clifton Road site adjacent to Emory University, covered seventeen separate disciplines, including bacteriology, toxicology, mycology, parasitology, virology, vector-borne diseases, and pathology. Here technicians could use electron microscopy to directly observe infected tissue, culture bacteria on appropriate media, and inoculate diseased material in cell cultures, eggs, and small laboratory animals. In addition, they could screen sputa and sera for antibodies to a range of antigens.

By the end of August, CDC technicians had scanned hundreds of tissue samples and used fluorescent antibodies against over a dozen different microbes. With the exception of one patient, who tested positive for mycoplasmal pneumonia, none of the sera showed significant antibody responses. Nor did tests of nasal and throat washings reveal the presence of chlamydia, *Y. pestis*, or more exotic bacteria and viruses, such as Lassa and Marburg. At one point, technicians got excited when three guinea pigs died of a mixed bacterial infection after inoculation with a lung suspension from a patient. However, it later transpired that the bacteria were typical of those found in patients after treatment with antibiotics or in postmortem overgrowth, and when the lung suspension was passed through a bacterial filter in an effort to exclude everything except a virus, it was no longer pathogenic for guinea pigs.* As the tests came up blank, the scientists tried different methods. One was to put blood samples in test tubes with antibodies against various microbes and look for a positive reaction. Mindful of the toxic chemicals theory, the scientists also subjected lung, liver, and kidney samples from deceased Legionnaires to radioactive assays for poisoning with twenty-three heavy metals, including mercury, arsenic, nickel, and cobalt.

After influenza and psittacosis, the next most likely suspect had been Q fever. Caused by *Coxiella burnetii*, an obligate intracellular parasite midway between a bacterium and a virus, Q fever used to be classed as a type of rickettsia. However, unlike other rickettsial diseases, such as typhus and Rocky Mountain spotted fever, which are transmitted by the bites of arthropods, humans typically get Q fever when they breathe in dust infected by contaminated animals (the principal animal reservoirs are cattle, sheep, and goats). Common symptoms are fever, severe headache, and a cough. In about half of patients, pneumonia ensues, and hepatitis is frequent enough that the combination of pneumonia and hepatitis is usually considered diagnostic. Unlike with typhus, a rash is rare and, though Q fever is an acute illness, patients usually recover even in the absence of antibiotics.

The researchers to whom it fell to test for Q fever were Charles Shepard, the head of the CDC's Leprosy and Rickettsia Branch, and his

---

* Many bacteria will continue to grow in tissue postmortem, hence the importance of embalming and cold storage to prevent putrefaction. However, most bacteria that cause disease cannot survive more than a few hours in a dead body.

assistant, Joe McDade. A bespectacled, blue-eyed scientist with a reputation for meticulous research, McDade had only just joined the CDC a
year earlier. Thirty-six years old, he had previously been stationed with
a Naval Medical Research Unit in North Africa, where he had worked
on rickettsial diseases. In theory, this made McDade the perfect person
for the job. However, at the time he had no experience of public health
microbiology and looked to Shepard and other more experienced CDC
hands for direction. After his overseas posting, McDade found the
work in Atlanta laborious and a little dull. Departing from standard
tests and other procedural deviations were not encouraged, he recalled.
Instead, he was expected to follow prescribed algorithms and testing
procedures, entering the results in a matrix that would hopefully line
up with the epidemiological evidence and bring about a resolution of
the mystery. Working with lung tissue from deceased Legionnaires,
McDade's first job was to grind up the autopsy material and inoculate it into guinea pigs. Q fever has an incubation period of a week
to ten days, so the next stage was to wait. If a guinea pig developed
fever, McDade euthanized the animal, removed some of its tissue, and
injected it into an embryonic egg. In this way, he hoped to obtain sufficient numbers of bacteria that could be stained and examined.

Part of the reason for McDade's lack of enthusiasm was that at the
time "everyone was looking for influenza or known causes of bacterial pneumonia," and there was no evidence that the Legionnaires
had been exposed to livestock, making Q fever highly unlikely. Sure
enough, when he inoculated the material into guinea pigs they developed fever within two or three days, far earlier than if the organism
had been *C. burnetti*. Modifying his procedure, McDade euthanized
the guinea pigs prematurely and removed a section of their spleens.
He then made impression smears on glass slides and stained them
to see what organisms he could observe through the microscope. At
the same time he used some of the tissue to prepare a suspension
and streaked it on an agar plate to see if anything would grow on

the media. Finally, he added antibiotics to the mixture to inhibit the growth of any contaminants that might be lurking in the tissue and inoculated the material directly into embryonated eggs so as to grow rickettsia should they be present.

He found no evidence of rickettsia; all the eggs remained perfectly healthy for more than ten days. Nor was he able to recover any bacteria from the agar plates. However, as he peered at the smears through the microscope, McDade would occasionally spot a rod-shaped, Gram-negative bacterium, "one here and another there." Distrusting his observations, McDade shared the slides with more experienced colleagues, only to be told that guinea pigs were "notoriously dirty animals" and what he had seen was most likely an "experimental contamination." "I was told there was an accumulating body of evidence that no bacteria were involved and what I had was an anomalous observation," he recalled. Instead, McDade was told to look for a virus.

As McDade and Shepard's efforts faltered, other scientists, abetted by politicians in Washington, revived the toxic metal and chemical contaminant theories. The leading advocate of the toxic metals theory was Dr. William F. Sunderman Jr., the head of laboratory medicine at the University of Connecticut School of Medicine. Early on in the outbreak, Sunderman and his father, William Sunderman Sr., professor of pathology at the Hahnemann Medical College, Philadelphia, had urged the public health authorities to collect urine and blood samples from suspected cases so they could be analyzed for toxic substances. The leading suspect in the Sundermans' view was nickel carbonyl. A colorless, odorless metal, nickel carbonyl is widely used in industrial operations and is highly toxic. Symptoms can present themselves anywhere from one to ten days after exposure and typically include a severe headache, dizziness, and muscle pains. In the first hour after exposure, victims may also complain of shortness of breath and a dry cough. Without treatment, exposure can result in acute pneumonitis and bronchopneumonia with high fever.

In mid-September, the younger Sunderman had studied six lung tissue samples from patients with Legionnaires' disease and found that five contained unusually high levels of nickel. However, while this suggested the patients may have inhaled a toxic substance, nickel concentrations in other tissues and organs, such as the liver and kidney, were normal. To exclude the possibility that the elevated readings were due to accidental contamination, he would also need to test urine and blood from Legionnaires, but unfortunately, in the confusion of the early days of the outbreak, public health officials had failed to collect and preserve specimens for future testing. Despite these caveats, at a congressional hearing in November chaired by John M. Murphy, a Democrat from Staten Island, New York, the Sundermans were highly critical of the CDC and the "flaws" in its investigation— flaws that they attributed to the "zeal" of public health authorities to see Congress enact legislation indemnifying vaccine manufacturers against prosecution arising from the swine flu immunization program. Sunderman Sr. was particularly critical, agreeing with a recent newspaper article in the *Washington Post* that had accused the CDC of "eagerness bordering on mania . . . to find swine flu in Pennsylvania." Indeed, in his congressional testimony, he went further than his son had been prepared to do, stating definitively that the outbreak *was* due to nickel carbonyl poisoning. Congressman Murphy was similarly critical, stating it was "inconceivable" that no one could say with any certainty whether the outbreak had been "murder; a virus; accidental introduction of a toxic substance; or a . . . convergence of factors yet to be determined." In particular, he described the lack of coordination between the CDC and other agencies as a national "embarrassment," telling House committee members that "nothing was done to search for toxic evidence until it was almost too late." Pointing out that "many experts [had] recognized the toxicological symptoms very early," he argued that the possibility of "foul play" could not be excluded and that toxic substances may have been placed on telephones, food, or the

Legionnaires' ice cubes. "It is entirely possible that a terrorist group or single fanatic might possess the technology to distribute a deadly poison or bacteria among a large group," he concluded.

It was not the first time Murphy had sought to stoke paranoia about the antiwar movement. In October, aides to his committee had leaked a story to the *Washington Post* saying that congressional investigators believed "a demented veteran or paranoid anti-military type" with some knowledge of chemistry may have been responsible for the Legionnaires' deaths. Such stories played to the suspicion and anxiety that infected American society in the mid-1970s which, arguably, has only become more pronounced with time. A decade earlier, historian Richard Hofstadter had coined the term *paranoid style* to describe "the sense of heated exaggeration, suspiciousness, and conspiratorial fantasy" he detected in extreme right-wing movements, such as the 1964 campaign for the White House by Barry Goldwater, the militantly anticommunist Republican senator from Arizona. By the 1970s, this paranoid style was arguably no longer confined to the Right, but following the assassination of leading lights of the civil rights movement, was also beginning to infect the Left, hence the popularity of theories blaming the deaths of Jack and Bobby Kennedy and Martin Luther King on the CIA, the Mafia, and the Ku Klux Klan, or some combination of all three.

The early 1970s was also a time of growing anxiety about nuclear energy and the dangers of environmental and chemical pollutants, such as Agent Orange, the highly toxic herbicide sprayed on the Vietnamese countryside, which was just beginning to give rise to cancers and other unexplained health problems among Vietnam vets and their children. As Laurie Garrett has argued, from the perspective of the Left, "events in Philadelphia fit neatly with the then vogue view that an unregulated chemical industry was raining toxic compounds upon the American people." By contrast, the Right was more inclined to view the outbreak as an act of sabotage, or as the Philadelphia Veterans of Foreign Wars put it, "a sneak attack against the finest kind of Americans."

This sense of moral panic did not escape Bob Dylan, who incorporated some of the wilder speculation into a song, "Legionnaires' Disease." Written for his touring guitarist, Billy Cross, the song opened with the verse: "Some say it was radiation, some say there was acid on the microphone / Some say a combination that turned their hearts to stone."

In retrospect this panic seems irrational, laughable even. After all, unlike cholera and plague, Legionnaires' disease was not contagious. Nor was it a disfiguring disease like smallpox, or one freighted with metaphors of waste and decay, like cancer and tuberculosis. On the other hand, the fact that its identity was unknown made it ripe for the projection of society's worst fears. Like Jack the Ripper, the mysterious killer had descended suddenly and unexpectedly on the Bellevue, then vacated the scene just as mysteriously. In the process, it had left few clues—or at least, none that the CDC's disease detectives had been able to parse—turning what was usually considered a safe and secure location into dangerous ground. It was a blow from which the Bellevue, already in financial trouble before the outbreak, would never recover. With newspapers using phrases like "mysterious and terrifying disease" and "the Philadelphia killer" to describe the outbreak, guests canceled their reservations one by one. The result was that on November 10, the management announced the Bellevue was no longer able "to withstand the economic impact of the worldwide, adverse publicity" and closed its doors to further business.

Not long after, Fraser decided it was also time for him to close the book on the EIS investigation and begin the laborious process of drafting his final report, known as an EPI-2. Despite going over the hotel with a fine-tooth comb and many hours of interviews, he was still no closer to identifying the pathogen or means of transmission. Privately, he was dismissive of the nickel carbonyl theory as the metal usually has an incubation period of less than thirty-six hours and rarely causes fevers above 101°F. Nor did he think it was food poisoning: the Legionnaires had purchased food from many different sources, and EIS officers had been unable to implicate a common meal at the convention. Similarly, although the cross-connection between the AHU and the Bellevue's potable water supply suggested a waterborne illness, more than one-third of the ill delegates insisted they had never drunk water at the hotel. By contrast, almost all the hotel employees, none of whom had suffered Legionnaires' disease, said they frequently drank from a fountain in the lobby.

In October, Fraser discussed the case with his boss, John V. Bennett. Bennett had been the lead investigator of the 1965 outbreak at St. Elizabeths Hospital. Based on the epidemiology of the outbreak (the cases were associated with proximity to open windows), Bennett had suspected airborne transmission. However, all attempts to identify the etiological agent had failed, so at the end of the investigation Bennett had filed the blood from St. Elizabeths patients in the CDC's serum banks in the hope that it might prove useful at a later date. "When you solve the Legionnaires' outbreak you will solve my outbreak at St. Elizabeths," he told Fraser.

Mulling over Bennett's words, Fraser thought an airborne agent might explain the sickness of both the Legionnaires and Broad Street pneumonia cases—individuals who had passed by the hotel without entering it. Fraser also noted the strong association between illness and time spent in the lobby, and the fact that after the convention a fault had been discovered in the AHU serving the lobby area, prompting the hotel's management to have the filters cleaned. This cleaning operation had taken place on August 6 and "may have inadvertently limited the ability of investigators to identify a toxic or microbiologic agent in the air handling system," Fraser wrote in his report. On the other hand, the relatively low attack rate "may rule against an airborne agent to some degree." All that Fraser could say with confidence is that the illness resembled an infectious disease and there had been no secondary spread. Unfortunately, despite exhaustive microbiological studies, all the tests had been negative. It was possible that as new tests and technologies became available, new toxins capable of causing pneumonitis might be discovered, but that lay in the future. At present, "no toxin is known that causes just this pattern of disease," he concluded, "and toxicological studies are also negative so far."

In all his years as an outbreak investigator Fraser had never come across a case quite like it; it stuck in the craw, but he had to admit defeat. So did Langmuir. The Philadelphia outbreak, he informed the press, constituted "the greatest epidemiological puzzle of the century."

CHAPTER V

LEGIONNAIRES' REDUX

"The discovery of the etiologic agent of Legionnaires' disease was accomplished in the face of overwhelming odds. All of the combined bacteriology and pathology experience accumulated since the beginning of the century pointed away from this agent being a bacterium."

—WILLIAM H. FOEGE, director, CDC, Senate Subcommittee on Health and Scientific Research, November 9, 1977

In a period when antibiotics and vaccines seemed to have closed the book on infectious disease, the Legionnaires' outbreak challenged medical confidence that America was on the brink of a germ-free era. Little wonder then that the CDC's failure to solve the puzzle of the century produced a lingering sense of insecurity and anxiety. However, outside of medical and public health circles, the same sense of anxiety did not attach to swine flu. This is odd when you consider that CDC officials had been warning of an epidemic since February. Indeed, in late March, President Ford had gone on television to drive home the concerns that an outbreak of swine flu was imminent. Flanked by the two godfathers of the polio vaccine, the scientists Albert Sabin and Jonas Salk, Ford told the American public that he had been advised that "there is a very real possibility that unless we take effective counteractions, there could be an epidemic of this dangerous disease next fall and winter." Accordingly, he was seeking a $135 million appropriation from Congress for sufficient vaccine "to inoculate every man, woman, and child in the United States."

Congress approved the appropriation bill in April, and by the middle of August had also passed legislation waiving corporate liability for the immunization campaign. Ironically, Congress's willingness to idemnify vaccine manufacturers had little to do with its enthusiasm for the insurance business and everything to do with the fears raised by the Philadelphia outbreak. Even though on August 5 Sencer had told senators he did not think the outbreak was due to swine flu, politicians were petrified he might be wrong and that they would end up being branded obstructionists who had impeded the delivery of a life-saving vaccine. Nonetheless, scientists' and politicians' enthusiasm for the flu immunization campaign was not shared by the public, with a Gallup poll in September indicating that only about half of all Americans were willing to be immunized. In other words, faced with a repeat of an epidemic on the scale of 1918, the public's response was to shrug its shoulders. This indifference turned to resistance when at the beginning of October the campaign finally got under way. Within ten days, one million Americans had rolled up their sleeves and received the jab, but on October 11 the campaign suffered a disastrous blow when it was reported that three elderly people in Pittsburgh, Pennsylvania, had died hours after having the inoculation. The deaths prompted a media scare that led to nine states suspending their vaccination programs. To calm the public's nerves and restore confidence, President Ford and his family were photographed receiving jabs at the White House. CDC scientists, meanwhile, attempted to educate the public, explaining that the risk of temporally associated deaths within forty-eight hours of inoculation occurred at a rate of 5/100,000 a day. By comparison, the anticipated death rate per day for *all* causes among citizens in Pennsylvania was 17/100,000. In other words, it was to be expected that some people would die after receiving the flu shot, but that did not mean there was a causal connection.

Unfortunately, by 1976 the public's unquestioning acceptance of scientific authority was beginning to wane, as were memories of life before vaccines against polio, measles, and other debilitating childhood diseases. Moreover, by now influenza experts in other countries were beginning to question the American scientific consensus that the swine flu isolated at Fort Dix was the harbinger of a new pandemic strain, a skepticism shared by WHO officials in Geneva who advocated a "wait and see" policy. As October turned to November with no signs of the feared pandemic, skepticism hardened. Still, the campaign might have been saved were it not for reports of cases of Guillain-Barré syndrome (GBS). A rare and occasionally lethal neurological syndrome, GBS occurs at a steady rate in the general population and, if a pandemic had been occurring, would have been deemed an acceptable risk. However, in the absence of a pandemic, the reports in December that as many as thirty people had developed the syndrome within a month of receiving the flu jab sparked widespread alarm, prompting the government to suspend the campaign so that the association with the vaccine could be investigated. The program was never restarted, and as cases of the syndrome soared—by the end of December, 526 cases were being reported, of which 257 had received the flu jab—the press and politicians in Washington began looking for a fall guy. The *New York Times* was especially harsh, labeling the campaign a "fiasco" and, in view of the fact that the pandemic had never materialized, a waste of time and effort. The result was that when Jimmy Carter moved into the White House in January, Joseph Califano Jr., the incoming secretary of Health, Education, and Welfare (HEW), demanded Sencer's resignation. Shamefully, Califano informed Sencer of his dismissal minutes before the pair were due to appear together at a meeting in Washington on the moratorium of the swine flu program. Worse, the whispered conversation in an HEW hallway was captured by the TV cameras, deepening Sencer's humiliation. According to public health historian George Dehner, this was "shabby treatment" for someone who had given sixteen years of service to the CDC, eleven as its director. On the other hand, Dehner writes, in his efforts to convince administration officials of the vaccination campaign's necessity, Sencer had deliberately downplayed the scientific uncertainty so as to give "a distorted vision of the new virus." The result was that "only the most dire vision of a swine flu pandemic remained."

Ironically, just three weeks before Sencer's very public firing, Shepard had rushed into his office to announce that he and McDade had solved the puzzle of the century. The culprit was a hitherto unknown Gram-negative bacterium. Other researchers had missed it because the bacterium was difficult to see using a conventional Gram stain. However, McDade had solved the problem using a different staining technique. According to Garrett, after all the pressure and frustration of the past year, Sencer was reluctant to accept what Shepard was telling him. "Shep, how sure are you?" "Better than ninety-five percent," he replied, "but I'd like to run a few more experiments before we go public."

There is an old saying in medical research: "fortune favours the prepared mind." The saying is usually attributed to Louis Pasteur, who famously stumbled on a vaccine against chicken cholera in 1880 when a colleague inoculated some chickens with an old culture of chicken cholera germs. In McDade's case, however, it was because he was a novice to public health microbiology and therefore not schooled in the same thought processes as his colleagues that a chance observation led him to the answer that had eluded them. It also helped that McDade was a worrier and a perfectionist. To his way of thinking, the peculiar rod-shaped bacteria he had weakly glimpsed through his microscope in August represented a loose end, and he didn't like it. However, it was not until late December that he thought to return to the problem. The impetus was a conversation with a man who had cornered him at a party shortly before Christmas. "I don't know how he knew I was CDC but he did," recalled McDade. "He said, 'We know you scientists are a little weird but we count on you and we're very disappointed.' I stuttered because I didn't know what to say. But it bothered me and stuck in my mind."

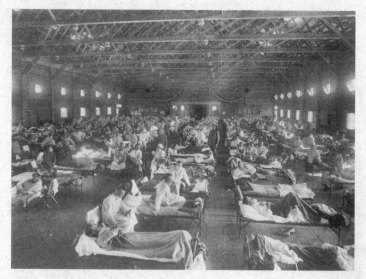

Emergency influenza ward: In March 1918 more than 1,200 soldiers were hopitalized when an influenza-like illness swept through Camp Funston at Fort Riley, Kansas. Some experts believe this was the herald of the spring wave of Spanish flu.

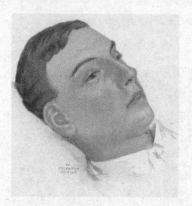

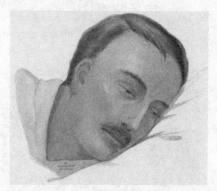

PLATE 1.—This illustrates an early case in which the facial colour is frankly red, and the patient might not appear ill were it not for the drooping of the upper eye-lids, giving a half-closed appearance to the eyes.

PLATE 2.—This illustrates a pronounced degree of the "heliotrope cyanosis." The patient is not in physical distress, but the prognosis is almost hopeless.

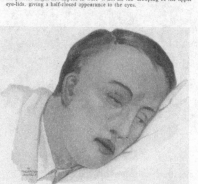

One of the key diagnostic signs of Spanish flu was heliotrope cyanosis, the three stages of which are shown here in an illustration by W. Thornton Shiells. Caused by deoxygenation of arterial blood as the lungs filled with choking fluids, the condition nearly always ended in death.

PLATE 3.—This illustrates another type of the cyanosis, in which the colour of the lips and ears arrests attention in contrast to the relative pallor of the face. The patient may yet live for twelve hours or more

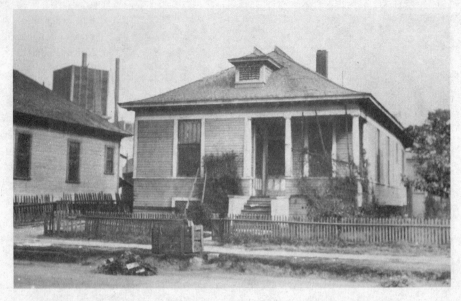

742 Clara Street: The so-called death house at the center of the 1924 pneumonic plague outbreak in the Mexican quarter of Los Angeles.

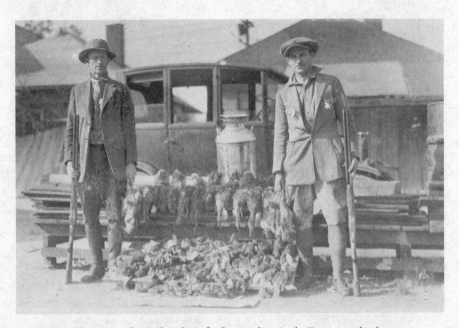

Squirrel hunters with one day's bag of 178 ground squirrels. To remove the threat of plague from downtown Los Angeles, the health department offered $1 for every dead squirrel or rat brought to its laboratory at Eighth Street.

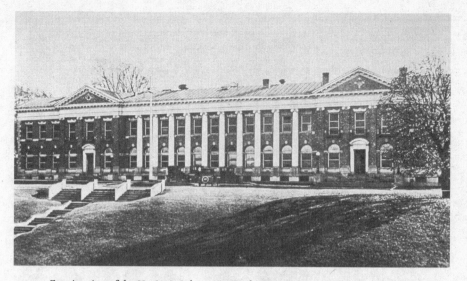

Exterior view of the Hygienic Laboratory, Washington, DC. Located at Twenty-Fifth Street and E Street NW, it was here that George McCoy conducted experiments on parrots infected with psittacosis in 1930.

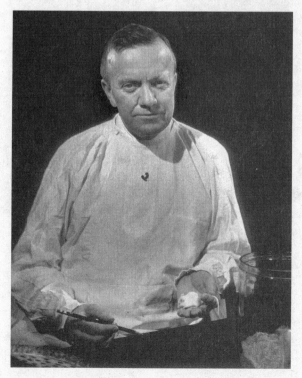

Charles Armstrong, pictured in his lab coat circa 1950, was one of the "heroes" of the parrot fever outbreak. After contracting the infection and recovering, his serum was used to treat the wife of an Idaho senator.

Bellevue-Stratford Hotel, Philadelphia: In the summer of 1976, the CDC recorded 182 cases of Legionnaires' disease following an American Legion convention at the hotel.

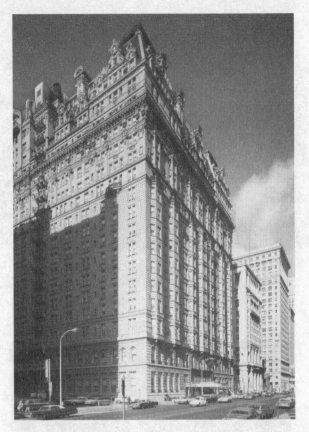

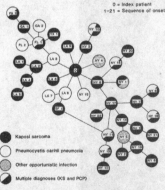

0 = Index patient
1–21 = Sequence of onset

● Kaposi sarcoma
○ Pneumocystis carinii pneumonia
◐ Other opportunistic infection
◑ Multiple diagnoses (KS and PCP)

City   LA – Los Angeles, NY – New York City, SF – San Francisco
State   FL – Florida, GA – Georiga, NJ – New Jersey, PA – Pennsylvania,
        TX – Texas

William Darrow's "cluster study" for the CDC tracing the sexual contacts of early homosexual male AIDS patients in southern California. Many people misread the "O," designating "Out[side]-of-California," as a zero, leading to Gaetan Dugas being erroneously dubbed "Patient Zero" of America's AIDS epidemic.

You won't get AIDS from everyday contact.
You won't get AIDS from being a friend.
You won't get AIDS from a mosquito bite.
You won't get AIDS from a kiss.
You won't get AIDS by talking.
You won't get AIDS by listening.
You won't get AIDS from a public pool.
You won't get AIDS from a pimple.
You won't get AIDS from a toilet seat.
You won't get AIDS from a haircut.
You won't get AIDS by donating blood.
You won't get AIDS from an airplane.
You won't get AIDS from tears.
You won't get AIDS from food.
You won't get AIDS from a hug.
You won't get AIDS from a towel.
You won't get AIDS from a telephone.
You won't get AIDS from a crowded room.

You won't get AIDS from an elevator.
You won't get AIDS from a greasy spoon.
You won't get AIDS from a bump.
You won't get AIDS by laughing.
You won't get AIDS by watching a movie.
You won't get AIDS from a cat.
You won't get AIDS from a schoolyard.
You won't get AIDS from going to a party.
You won't get AIDS from taking a trip.
You won't get AIDS from a dog bite.
You won't get AIDS from visiting a city.
You won't get AIDS from a cab.
You won't get AIDS from a bus.
You won't get AIDS at a play.
You won't get AIDS by dancing.
You won't get AIDS because someone is
different from you.
You won't get AIDS from a classroom.

Stop Worrying About How You Won't Get AIDS. And Worry About How You Can.

You *can* get AIDS from sexual intercourse
with an infected partner.
You *can* get AIDS from sharing drug
needles with an infected person.
You *can* get AIDS by being born to an
infected mother.

AMERICA
RESPONDS
TO AIDS

"Stop Worrying About How You Won't Get AIDS. And Worry About How You Can.": A CDC poster from the early 1980s correcting popular misconceptions about the transmission of HIV.

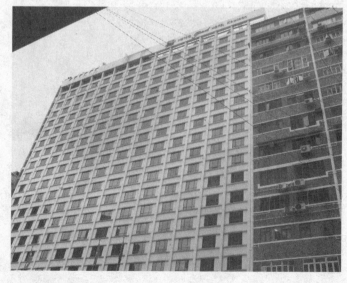

View of the Metropark Kowloon on Waterloo Road, Hong Kong. In February 2003, sixteen guests at the hotel, then known as the Metropole, were infected with SARS after a Chinese professor who was incubating the virus checked in.

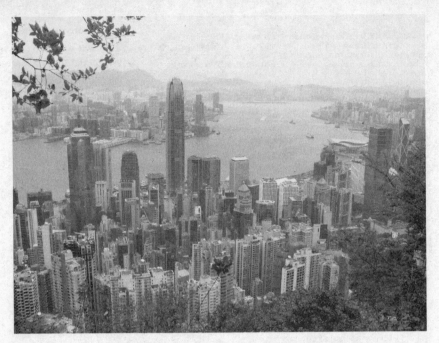

Hong Kong is one of the most densely populated cities in the world. Its proximity to Guangdong in southern China makes it a "sentinel" for new strains of bird flu and other emerging infectious diseases.

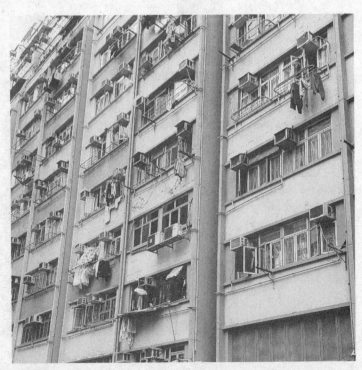

A typical Hong Kong street scene showing multiple occupancy apartments. The average Hong Kong adult has just two square meters of living space.

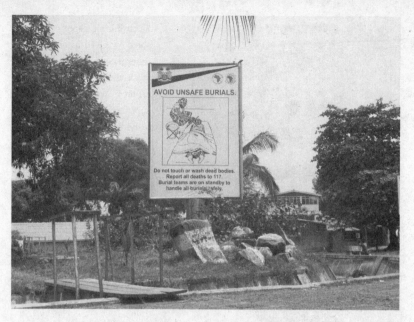

"Avoid Unsafe Burials": Public health messaging on a roundabout in Aberdeen, a suburb of Freetown, Sierra Leone, warning people of the dangers of touching or washing the bodies of Ebola victims.

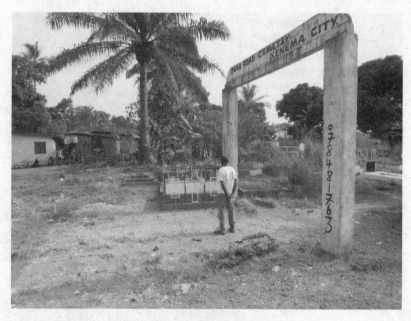

Mohamed Sow, a driver for Tulane's Lassa Fever research program, visits the grave of Mbalu J. Fonnie at Dama Road Cemetery in Kenema, Sierra Leone. Fonnie was one of eleven nurses who died when Ebola ripped through wards of Kenema General Hospital in July and August 2014.

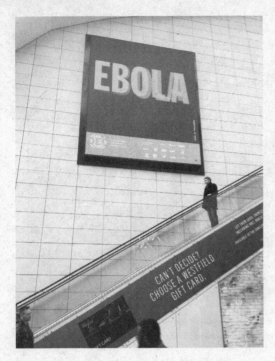

Electronic sign sponsored by the Disasters Emergency Committee at Westfield shopping center in West London appealing for donations to aid the medical and humanitarian relief effort for Ebola in West Africa.

"Danger – Shark Zone": A sign on the beach at Boa Viagem near Recife in northeastern Brazil warning bathers to avoid swimming at high tide and other times when sharks are active. Recife was also one of the cities hardest hit by the Zika epidemic.

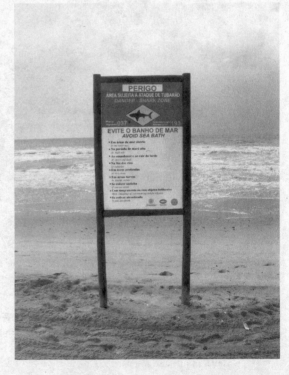

It had always been McDade's habit to use the week between Christ-mas and New Year's to resolve any outstanding paperwork in prepara-tion for the new working year. While tidying his office he spotted the glass slides with the smears he had taken from the guinea pigs in a box on the shelf and decided to have another look. The exercise, he recalled, was like "searching for a missing contact lens on a basket-ball court with your eyes four inches away from the floor." Eventually, however, McDade spotted a cluster of organisms in the corner of one of the microscopic fields. To McDade's way of thinking, the fact that the organisms were clustered together "suggested that it wasn't just organisms that happened to be there but were actually growing there inside the guinea pig." It was at this point that McDade decided to have another go at culturing the organism. His thinking was "if I can rule out that it has nothing to do with the disease my conscience will be salved and I can go about my business." It was at this point that McDade's expertise as a rickettsial specialist and his willingness to depart from conventional patterns of thought came into play. Going to the freezer drawers containing spleen tissue from suspect guinea pigs that had been put on ice in August, McDade thawed the samples and inoculated some of the tissue into embryonated eggs. However, this time he withheld antibiotics in order to allow whatever organ-isms were present in the guinea pig tissue to grow freely. Five to seven days later the eggs died and McDade took new smears. As before, he applied a Gimenez stain, a technique which had been developed spe-cifically for rickettsial organisms, and, once again, spotted the same rod-shaped bacteria growing in clusters. Could these bacteria be responsible for the guinea pigs' deaths, and could the same bacteria be responsible for the Legionnaires' disease outbreak? To answer the question, McDade retrieved some preserved serum from the Legion-naires' cases and mixed it with the organism he had found in the eggs. If a patient's serum contained antibodies specific to the organism, an observable reaction would take place. It did. "They just lit up dramatically," he said. "My neck hair bristled. I wasn't sure what I'd got there but I knew it was something."

McDade immediately shared his findings with Shepard, and together they ran further tests using paired serum samples taken from Legionnaires two or more weeks apart. If it could be shown that the reaction took place at much higher dilution in the second serum sample than in the first, this would be strong evidence that the patient had recently recovered from the disease caused by the organism. At the same time, McDade and Shepard repeated the test using blinded samples from both Legionnaires' and non-Legionnaires' patients, some of whom had had other pneumonias or were healthy. Nearly fifty years later, McDade vividly recounted the moment of discovery:

> When we'd finished all the tests, later that evening, they brought down the paper and we broke the code. All the normal specimens from healthy people were negative, specimens from patients with other pneumonias were all negative. Then we looked at the Legionnaires' disease specimens. Specimens taken from Legionnaires early in the illness had little or no antibodies, and specimens taken later in illness had very high levels of antibody, which suggested they had been infected with this bacteria. So that was the moment when we knew we'd found the etiologic agent.

When Shepard informed Sencer of the breakthrough he could hardly contain his excitement and insisted that they issue an announcement in the next edition of the *Morbidity and Mortality Weekly Report*, the CDC's house journal, and schedule a press conference for the same day, January 18, 1977. This was earlier than Shepard and McDade had been anticipating—normally, scientific discoveries take several months to be written up before being submitted to a scientific journal. Because of the political pressure on Sencer, however, he could not wait for the usual peer review process. Worried that they would be laughing stocks if their methodology was subsequently found to be faulty, Shepard and McDade double-checked their results. Then, out of curiosity, McDade decided to look in the CDC's stores for serum from other unsolved outbreaks. That's when he came across the stored blood from the patients at St. Elizabeths Hospital. McDade injected the blood into chicken eggs, then added the organism he had isolated in Philadelphia. The eggs lit up immediately, indicating that there was an antibody reaction and that the St. Elizabeths patients had been infected with the same organism. Bennett's intuition had been correct: in solving the Philadelphia outbreak, Fraser and his team had also solved the mystery of the earlier outbreak in Washington, DC.

News of Shepard and McDade's discovery traveled around the world, prompting scientists at other research establishments in Europe and elsewhere to duplicate the CDC's results. As scientists exchanged information and examined old case files, it became apparent that St. Elizabeths was not the only prior outbreak of Legionnaires' disease. Blood specimens from patients at the Oakland County Health Department in Pontiac, Michigan, in 1968 also tested positive for antibodies to *Legionella pneumophila*, as the organism was now known, suggesting that they had been infected by the same agent, though why there had been no pneumonia in the "Pontiac Fever" cases and why the outbreak had not resulted in any fatalities was unclear. That was not all: in May 1977, Marilyn Bozeman, a rickettsia specialist at the Walter Reed Army Institute of Research, in Bethesda, Maryland, informed McDade that she had seen very similar organisms in guinea pigs while investigating specimens taken from an outbreak in 1959. Like McDade, she had assumed these were contaminants and described them as "rickettsia-like." It was only later, when she ran new tests, that she found they were actually two new species of *Legionella*, *Legionella bozemanii* and *Legionella micdadei*. It was subsequently found that *L. micdadei* had also been responsible for an outbreak of "Fort Bragg fever" in 1943 and that Walter Reed also had an isolate of *L. pneumophila* dating from 1947.

Then, in early summer, came news of an outbreak at a medical center in Burlington, Vermont. EIS officers rushed to the scene, and by September they had documented sixty-nine cases of Legionnaires' disease. However, once again, the source of the exposure eluded them. Soon, there were reports of other outbreaks in hospitals across the United States. The most notable was an outbreak that began at the Wadsworth Medical Center, a veterans' hospital in Los Angeles, in the summer and which by the end of the year had claimed sixteen lives. At around the same time, a smaller epidemic broke out at a hospital in Nottingham, England, sickening fifteen people. Once again, no common source was found, but two of the sera from patients sent to the CDC for analysis tested positive for antibodies to *Legionella*. That was not all: in 1978 CDC scientists confirmed that *Legionella* had been responsible for a mysterious outbreak of pneumonia at the Rio Park hotel in Benidorm, Spain, that had been blamed for the deaths of three Scottish holiday-makers five years earlier. The result was that when, in 1980, another outbreak occurred at the same hotel, epidemiologists took water samples and found the bacterium lurking in the showerheads. Apparently, an old water well had been brought back into use five days before the start of the outbreak and had fed water infected with *L. pneumophila* directly into the hotel. Investigators concluded that those who showered and washed first thing each morning were at most risk because the bacteria multiplied overnight in water standing in peripheral pipe work. In all, a total of fifty-eight people were sickened, and one woman died. Like the outbreak at the Bellevue, the Rio Park outbreak sparked considerable press interest and inspired the thriller writer Desmond Bagley to pen a novel, *Bahama Crisis* (1980), in which a Caribbean holiday resort's water system is deliberately seeded with *Legionella* bacteria in an act of industrial espionage.

By now, it was becoming clear that Legionnaires' disease was closely associated with hotels, hospitals, and other large buildings. But though it was suspected that cooling towers and modern air conditioning systems facilitated the spread of the organism, attempts to isolate *L. pneumophilia* from the cooling towers of hospitals failed. Then, in 1978 came a breakthrough with the report of an outbreak in the heart of Manhattan's garment district. By September, the CDC had identified seventeen cases, the majority of them centered around a building on 35th Street between Seventh Avenue and Broadway. On the CDC's advice, the city ordered businesses in the immediate vicinity to switch off their air conditioners. The agency then collected epidemiological samples from nearby buildings, including the cooling tower on the roof of Macy's Department Store located directly opposite the building on 35th Street. The sample tested positive for *Legionella*, but the CDC did not have sufficient epidemiological evidence to say the Macy's cooling tower was to blame. However, earlier that year, investigators had attended another outbreak at the Indiana Memorial Union and recovered *L. pneumophila* from the Union's cooling tower, so it was pretty obvious that cooling towers were responsible for many of the outbreaks. In addition, scientists found a nearby stream teeming with other species of the same bacteria, suggesting that the organism was widespread in the environment.

Currently, the genus *Legionella* comprises nearly forty different species and sixty-one serogroups.* However, it is one species, *L. pneumophila*, that is responsible for 90 percent of Legionnaires' disease cases. A facultative intracellular parasite, it is unable to grow outside of cells. Instead, it has evolved to live in natural aquatic environments, such as lakes, streams, ponds, and ground water. These environments are teeming with amoeba and protozoa that routinely ingest other ubiquitous bacteria as food. However, legionellae are able to evade these microbial processes and "trick" the amoeba into ingesting

---

* A serogroup is a group of bacteria that share a common antigen.

them. Once inside an amoeba, the bacterium multiplies intracellularly before releasing dozens of newly formed legionellae into the water. The new organisms then try to trick other amoebae into ingesting them. In this way, legionellae are considered "Trojan horse" bacteria.

Under natural conditions, water rarely reaches the temperatures necessary for the bacteria to multiply (legionellae grow best at temperatures of 72°F to 113°F), ensuring that populations are kept to safe levels. Man-made environments are different, however. Hotels, hospitals, and other large buildings are home to a number of devices that utilize water at ideal temperatures for the growth of *Legionella* bacteria. These include showerheads, hot tubs, whirlpool spas, water fountains, humidifiers, misting equipment, and architectural fountains. Cooling towers are of particular concern because the pools of warm water are open to the atmosphere—indeed, *Legionella* bacteria have been repeatedly isolated from the biofilms of slime and encrusted sludge on top of such towers, with some surveys indicating that as many as half of all cooling towers in the United States may be contaminated with the organisms. If such towers are not regularly serviced, this contaminated water can be aerosolized into microscopic droplets containing *Legionella*, enabling the organism to be drawn directly into a person's lungs. One way this may occur is during the cooling process, when warm water from the condenser or chiller unit is sprayed across the fill at the top of a cooling tower, splintering the water into tiny droplets. While most of the water returns to the collecting pan to be circulated to the heat source to cool refrigerant from the air conditioning unit, some of the water is aerosolized, resulting in the production of a fine mist at the top of the tower. If a drift eliminator is not fitted to the tower or the eliminator is inadequate, this mist may then be drawn into nearby air intake vents and air shafts. Under certain temperature conditions, the mist can also cascade down the side of the building to ground level, from where it may be drawn in through open windows or inhaled by passing pedestrians. A third possible route of contamination is the pipework supplying potable water to showers and so forth, especially where hot water systems are run intermittently and water is left to stand for long periods in pipes. Finally, in theory, contamination can also occur if there is a direct link from the water tower to the chilled water supply of an air conditioning unit.

One reason *Legionella* is so dangerous is that the same strategy that enables the organism to evade ingestion by amoebae also enables the organism to escape attack by the alveolar macrophages, the body's first line of defense against lung infections. Instead, legionellae multiply within the cells of the alveoli, before spilling out and colonizing other lung cells. If other host defense responses are not activated in time, the result is pneumonia and systemic illness.

In the United States, the incidence of Legionnaires' disease varies from state to state, with the highest incidence being recorded in the summer and fall. Those aged sixty and over are at greatest risk, especially if they suffer from chronic lung disease or have other underlying medical conditions. The disease also occurs more frequently in men than women, though whether this is due to the higher prevalence of cigarette smoking and lung disease in men, or some other predisposing factor, is not known (cigarette smokers have a two- to fourfold higher risk of developing Legionnaires' disease than nonsmokers). Hospitals present a particular risk because of inadequate servicing of hot water systems and the way that such settings bring together large numbers of immunocompromised patients. Confined to their beds for long periods in wards, these patients, many of whom may be suffering from other conditions and have compromised immune systems, present the organism with the ideal host. Surveys have also found that modern medical technologies such as immunosuppressive therapies, intubation, anesthesia, and the placing of nasogastric tubes, also increase the risk of pneumonias due to Legionnaires' disease.

In 1978, the CDC held an international meeting to review what had been learned about *Legionella*, its epidemiology, and its ecology.

By now, McDade had perfected a technique for visualizing the organism using a special silver stain that colored the walls of the Gram-negative bacteria. Meanwhile, other researchers were learning how to cultivate it on charcoal yeast agar, a special medium supplemented with iron and cysteine. In addition, using a fluorescent-antibody staining technique, CDC researchers had demonstrated that organisms observed by pathologists in lung tissue recovered from Legionnaires in Philadelphia were in fact *L. pneumophila*. Unfortunately, however, the final piece of evidence—legionellae from the water tower on the roof of the Bellevue—eluded investigators as the hotel had now been closed and the tower and the air conditioning units thoroughly cleaned. Nevertheless, in light of the outbreaks seen at hospitals and other buildings in the United States, Fraser had little doubt that the hotel's water tower had been to blame. Noting that the convention had coincided with a marked temperature inversion in Philadelphia, he speculated that this inversion could have caused mist from the tower to come across the edge of the roof and "cascade down the side of the building." In this way, the contaminated air could have enveloped people on the sidewalk and been sucked into the lobby through a vent near the ground floor, thus accounting for both the cases observed among delegates and the Broad Street pneumonias. There were two further pieces of evidence implicating the Bellevue. The first was the discovery of antibodies to *Legionella* in eleven members of another convention group that had visited the hotel two years earlier and whose members had suffered similar fevers and pneumonias. The second was a survey of hotel staff who had been employed at the hotel at around the same time. They also had antibodies to *Legionella*. This suggested that hotel staff had been exposed from time to time and had managed to acquire immunity, which was why so few of them had succumbed to the infection in 1976. By contrast, the Legionnaires had no such history of exposure.

⊰≋≻

THE LEGIONNAIRES' DISEASE outbreak is a classic example of how new technologies and changes to the built environment designed to improve hygiene and ameliorate the conditions of life are constantly giving rise to new threats to health and well-being. It also illustrates how, in certain political and cultural contexts, epidemics that might otherwise have gone unnoticed can command wide public attention and provoke considerable anxiety.

L. pneumophila has been around for millennia, but it was not until we began building cities and equipping buildings with indoor plumbing and hot water systems that we presented the bacterium with a new ecological niche in which to prosper. And it was not until we added other luxuries, such as air conditioning, showers, humidifiers, and misters, that we gave the bacterium an efficient way to aerosolize and colonize the human respiratory tract. Even so, it took several years for doctors and public health experts to wake up to the pathogenic threat posed by the presence of this ancient organism in the heart of modern metropolises.

One reason is that prior to the invention of a method for culturing the bacterium and diagnosing Legionella infections, Legionnaires' disease was indistinguishable from other atypical pneumonias for which a causative agent had yet to be identified. This made it largely invisible to physicians and respiratory disease experts who believed that pneumonia was mostly a problem of the past. Even where outbreaks were sufficiently unusual to draw the attention of doctors and public health experts, as had been the case at St. Elizabeths Hospital in 1965 and Pontiac, Michigan in 1968, investigations were inconclusive and had reached dead ends. This might also have been the fate of the CDC's inquiry into the outbreak at the Bellevue. That it was not is due, first, to its occurrence at a time of acute national anxiety about another epidemic disease, and second, to the intense media interest in the outbreak, sparked both by the focus on swine flu and by the fact that the victims were a venerated and vulnerable section of the American population. However, for all the resources at the CDC's disposal, in the final analysis these factors might have counted for nothing had it not been for the determination of one scientist and his willingness to set aside preconceived notions and patterns of thought.

By 1976, medical researchers were confident that they had identified all the leading causes of pneumonia and that, in any case, the condition responded to treatment with penicillin or one of the new generation of antibiotics, such as erythromycin and rifampicin. What few realized was that only half of sporadic pneumonia cases could be determined with existing diagnostic tests, much less that there had been several outbreaks for which a causal agent had never been identified. When examining pathology specimens and bacterial cultures, laboratory technicians had been taught to look, first, for the pneumococcus and, if that was absent, other *known* bacterial and mycobacterial causes of the disease. Using long-established culturing and staining techniques, it was possible to grow these bacteria on laboratory media and then color them with Gram stains or other common dyes. But what of an organism that could not be cultivated on the usual media and which, because it lacked a cell wall, could not be easily visualized with existing stains either? What, in other words, of an *unknown unknown*? This was the problem that confronted McDade when, using a stain developed for rickettsia, he peered through his microscope and spotted a faint rod-shaped organism growing in clusters. Because the organism did not conform to any of the known bacterial causes of pneumonia, McDade's colleagues insisted it must be a "contaminant." That is what their experience of cultivating bacteria in guinea pigs and their microbiology training had taught them. By contrast, McDade's mind was unprepared by previous experience for such an observation, and the more he ruminated on it the more he became concerned. What if it was the stain and not experimental error that had brought the bacteria to light, and what if his observation was not an anomaly? Thus it was that a chance observation led McDade in the direction opposite to that of his colleagues and to an eventual resolution of the problem.

Legionnaires' disease also illustrates the role of medical technology and human behavior in shaping our interactions with pathogens. It was not simply that water towers and air conditioning systems afforded an old bacterium a new place in which to breed; to provoke an outbreak, the bacterium also had to meet a group of highly susceptible individuals. This happened first at hospitals and medical centers, where the expansion in intensive care beds in the 1960s and the growing number of elderly or mentally ill patients receiving institutional treatment increased the bacterium's chances of finding an appropriate host. However, it also occurred at meatpacking plants and other large industrial premises with chiller units. And, of course, it also happened at luxury hotels and other large buildings with cooling towers and state-of-the-art air conditioning systems. The Bellevue was not alone in installing a Carrier refrigeration unit in the 1950s. In 1952, in preparation for that year's Republican and Democratic conventions, engineers from the Carrier Company brought air conditioning to the International Amphitheatre in Chicago. Six years later, Carrier installed similar units in the Fidelity Building in Los Angeles, making it the first fully air-conditioned office building in California. By the end of the decade, air conditioning had also arrived in domestic homes, fueling migration to Florida and other "Sun Belt" states. The result was that by 1969, when Carrier announced that the towers of New York's World Trade Center would be cooled and heated by its equipment, no American office or home, large or small, was considered complete without air conditioning.

At the time, of course, no one realized that cooling towers and air conditioners presented an infectious disease risk. This only became significant *after* January 1977, when Joe McDade's isolation of *L. pneuomophila* resulted in the discovery of the organism in other buildings across the United States. Once *L. pneuomophila* had been identified, researchers were able to show it submitted to treatment with erythromycin and rifampicin, drugs that quickly became the standard therapy. The result is that today legionellae are recognized around the world as an important cause of community-acquired pneumonia outbreaks, prompting routine checks on the cooling towers of hotels and hospitals. That is not to say the threat has disappeared: despite the wider availability of diagnostic tests, legionellae are thought to be responsible for around 2 percent of pneumonia cases in the United States annually (around 50,000 cases). Moreover, outbreaks continue to occur with disturbing regularity wherever public water management standards or the inspection and cleaning of private water towers is found wanting. For instance, between 2014 and 2015, ninety people in Flint, Michigan, contracted Legionnaires' disease and twelve died after the town switched its water source from Detroit's system to the Flint River. And in 2015, New York City experienced the largest Legionnaires' outbreak in its history when the organism sickened 133 people living in apartment blocks in the South Bronx, killing 16. It later transpired that the source of the outbreak was a hotel water tower teeming with *Legionella* bacteria. In the most recent period for which figures are available—2000 to 2014—the CDC recorded almost a threefold increase in cases of legionellosis, which comprises both Legionnaires' disease and Pontiac fever, across the United States. Of these, 5,000 cases a year were due to Legionnaires' alone and the mortality rate was 9 percent. Of course, not all these outbreaks were the result of poorly maintained water systems or aging plumbing. America's aging population, the wider availability of diagnostic tests, and more reliable reporting to local and state health departments and the CDC most likely also played a role. A further factor may be climate change: as summers become hotter and unseasonably warm temperatures continue into the fall, the more likely it is that plumes of contaminated water will issue from water towers unless effective chlorination and other disinfectant measures are taken. Unfortunately, all too frequently, they are not.

To the extent that Legionnaires' disease tapped into Cold War fears about biological weapons and chemical toxins, it seemed to hark back to the preoccupations of the 1950s; hence, Congress's concern that it was a "missed alarm." But to the extent that it was a disease completely new to medical science, and one that could be traced to new technologies and alterations to the built environment, it seemed to represent a new paradigm of public health, one that would become increasingly relevant in the closing decades of the twentieth century. Indeed, by 1994, with the publication of Laurie Garrett's *The Coming Plague*, Legionnaires' disease was being seen as one of a series of "emerging infectious diseases" (EIDs), whose appearance was threatening to undo the medical advances of the postwar years and, with it, the certitude that advanced industrialized societies no longer needed to fear the plagues that had bedeviled previous eras. That the outbreak in Philadelphia in 1976 had coincided with the emergence the same year of a new viral hemorrhagic fever at a remote mission hospital in Yambuku, Zaire, close to the Ebola River, only served to underline these parallels; hence, the disease's inclusion in an iconic list of EIDs drawn up by the Institute of Medicine in 1992. The authors' biggest concern, however, was not Legionnaires' disease or Ebola, but HIV, a previously unknown virus that had first become visible to medical science in around 1981, and which by 1992 was recognized as the agent of one of the largest pandemics in history.

CHAPTER VI

AIDS IN AMERICA, AIDS IN AFRICA

"This is a very, very dramatic illness. I think we can say,
quite assuredly, that it is new."

—JAMES CURRAN, epidemiologist, 1982

I n December 1980, Dr. Michael Gottlieb was looking for an unusual teaching case to present to residents at the University of California Medical Center Los Angeles (UCLA) when one of his colleagues stumbled on a patient named Michael. A thirty-three-year-old artist, Michael had been admitted to the emergency room suffering from extreme weight loss and looked like an anorexic. In addition, his mouth was full of thrush, or candidiasis, a yeast infection usually seen in patients with weakened immune systems. Intrigued, Gottlieb, then a young assistant professor specializing in immunology, led residents to Michael's bedside and afterwards discussed the case with them. "There was something medically interesting about him," Gottlieb recalled. "He *smelled* like an immune deficiency."

Gottlieb's intuition was correct: Michael's antibody-producing capacity seemed to be intact, but when a colleague ran a specialized test using the latest monoclonal antibody technology he discovered that Michael had very few T cells. In particular, he found that a subset of Michael's T cells, known as CD4 cells, were perilously low. The central controllers of the immune system, CD4 cells are required for every type of immune response—whether to signal CD8 "killer" cells, whose job it is to destroy virus-infected cells; activate macrophages, a type of white blood cell that patrols for pathogens; or alert B lymphocytes, which produce antibodies against foreign invaders. Once these CD4 cells have been eliminated, sooner or later the entire immune system crashes. Their absence almost certainly explained the thrush. According to Gottlieb, the yeast infection was so extensive that Michael's mouth looked as if it was full of "cottage cheese." But it was impossible to arrive at a definitive diagnosis, so Michael was discharged. However, within a week he had developed pneumonia and had to be readmitted.

Concerned that Michael might have contracted an opportunistic lung infection, Gottlieb convinced a pulmonary specialist to perform a bronchoscopy and send a sample of his lung tissue to the laboratory. To Gottlieb's surprise, the tissue came back positive for *Pneumocystis carinii pneumonia*, or PCP, a rare fungal infection seen almost exclusively in malnourished newborns and infants in intensive care, terminally ill cancer patients, or the recipients of organ transplants. What such patients shared in common was compromised immune systems. For a young man to develop PCP was practically unheard of. "It was a distinctly unusual thing for someone previously healthy to walk into a hospital so significantly ill. It just didn't fit any recognized disease or syndrome that we were aware of." By March, Michael had been hospitalized, but no amount of drugs or experimental therapies would arrest the progress of the infection, and in May 1981 he died. The autopsy found *pneumocystis* throughout his lungs. Later, trying to figure out what could have caused Michael's immune system to give up on him, Gottlieb reviewed the artist's medical charts and saw that he had a cornucopia of sexually transmitted diseases (STDs). He also recalled a conversation in which Michael had mentioned that he was gay, but then Los Angeles had long boasted a sizable gay community, so it was difficult to see what bearing this could have on the matter.

Gottlieb was not the only doctor in Los Angeles to spot an unusual constellation of symptoms in gay men that fall and winter. The previous October, Joel Weisman, a local physician with a largely gay practice, had also treated two men for thrush. In addition, the men had chronic fevers and suffered from diarrhea and lymphadenopathy— swollen lymph nodes. In February one of the men's symptoms worsened and he was admitted to UCLA, where Gottlieb tested his blood and found the same abnormality that Michael had: a lower than expected number of CD4 cells. Soon after, he also developed PCP, as did the second patient in Weisman's care. In addition, both men had active cytomegalovirus (CMV), a type of herpes virus which is spread in bodily fluids, typically through kissing and sex, and which is usually quiescent in healthy adults. By April Gottlieb was becoming sufficiently concerned to call a former student, Wayne Shandera, now a member of the CDC's Epidemic Intelligence Service in Los Angeles. Gottlieb told Shandera of his suspicion that there was a new disease circulating in Los Angeles and asked him to check the LA County health records for other reports of PCP and/or CMV. Shandera quickly located a report about a man in Santa Monica who had recently been diagnosed with *Pneumocystis* and was deathly ill in the hospital. Soon after Shandera's visit, the man died and, on autopsy, CMV was found in his lungs.

Unbeknownst to Gottlieb and Weisman, by now physicians in New York were also seeing similar cases of swollen lymph nodes, low CD4 cell counts, and PCP in gay men in their care. At autopsy many were also found to be infected with CMV. Observing these patients up close was a shocking experience. Donna Mildvan, chief of infectious disease at Beth Israel Hospital, New York, recorded how in one case involving a German man who had formerly worked as a chef in Haiti and who had died in December, she had cultured CMV directly from his eyeball. "We were totally bewildered. . . . I can't even begin to tell you what an awful experience it was." Dr. Alvin Friedman-Kien, a dermatologist and virologist at New York University's Medical Center, was similarly disturbed to find that many of the patients also had Kaposi's sarcoma (KS), an extremely rare type of skin cancer typically seen in elderly Jewish men or men of eastern European and Mediterranean descent. Most dermatologists might go their whole career and see only one case of KS, but by February Friedman-Kien was aware of twenty cases of KS in the New York area alone. One of the most heartbreaking involved a young Shakespearian actor who presented at Friedman-Kien's practice in January with pink-purple spots on his face. The spots were so extensive, Friedman-Kien recalled, "he couldn't cover them up anymore."

In medicine, as in other professions, being first is everything—no one remembers the second person to describe a new disease—and by June Gottlieb was ready to go into print, informing the editor of the *New England Journal of Medicine* that he had "possibly a bigger story than Legionnaires' Disease." By now Gottlieb had five severe pneumonia cases (the fifth had come to him via a Beverley Hills physician). All were gay men between the ages of twenty-nine and thirty-six, all had PCP, candidiasis, and CMV, and three had low CD4 cell counts (in the two others, immune deficiency had not been studied). In addition, Gottlieb and Weisman noted, all five had also used "poppers"—amyl nitrate or butyl nitrate inhalers so named for the noise the ampules make when broken. However, their leading hypothesis at this stage was that the disease was due to CMV and, perhaps, some other virus, such as Epstein-Barr, interacting with one another so as to compromise the immune system. From a public health point of view this was worrying. Sexual health clinics across the United States had recently seen a marked increase in CMV cases which, along with other sexually transmitted diseases, such as hepatitis B and gonorrhea, were running at epidemic levels in the gay community.

Given the interest in getting the announcement out quickly, the editor of the *New England Journal of Medicine* advised Gottlieb to submit a brief article to the CDC's Sexually Transmitted Diseases division for publication in the agency's house journal, *Morbidity and Mortality Weekly Report*, on the understanding that the *New England Journal of Medicine* would consider a longer article at a later date. Jim Curran, the official who headed the STD division, immediately recognized the article's significance, not least because he was concerned about the recent increase in STDs in gay men and had been working closely with the homosexual community to evaluate the risk factors for hepatitis B. Before publishing the article, however, he asked a female colleague to check whether there had been any other reports of PCP in people without cancer, or who had not received organ transplants and had been taking drugs to suppress their immune systems. Looking back over fifteen years, she could find only one such case. Alarmingly, however, orders for pentamidine, an anti-PCP drug that was no longer in commercial production and for which the CDC had a small emergency stock, had jumped from the usual fifteen requests a year to thirty in the first five months of 1981. Curran did not require further convincing, and on June 5, 1981, he published Gottlieb's article in the *Morbidity and Mortality Weekly Report* together with an accompanying editorial. Noting that PCP was almost exclusively limited to severely immunosuppressed patients, Curran commented that its occurrence in previously healthy individuals was "unsettling," and the fact that all five individuals were gay suggested "an association between some aspect of a homosexual lifestyle or disease acquired through sexual contact and *Pneumocystis* pneumonia in this population." Although no definite conclusion could be reached about the role of CMV infections, Curran also noted recent surveys showing that many homosexual men carried CMV in their semen and that "seminal fluid may be an important vehicle of CMV transmission." In other words, there was no evidence that CMV was the cause of the mysterious new syndrome, but sexual transmission was suspected. Though hedged with qualifications, Curran's conclusion was prophetic: "All the above observations suggest the possibility of a cellular-immune dysfunction related to a common exposure that predisposes individuals to opportunistic infections such as pneumocystis and candidiasis." No one could have imagined that within months of that article appearing, these strange symptoms would be the talk of Hollywood, and by the following summer the world would have learned a terrifying new acronym. Curran may not have realized it but he had just described AIDS, acquired immunodeficiency syndrome.

IN THE FORTY YEARS SINCE—the CDC settled on the acronym in 1982—public attitudes toward AIDS have gone from indifference, to horror and dread, to seeing it as just another infectious disease, one that can be treated with an arsenal of drugs that suppress but never quite eliminate the human immunodeficiency virus (HIV), which is the cause of the immune deficiency that allows the opportunistic infections with which AIDS is associated to occur. In this transition from fear to familiarity, it is easy to forget the shocking sight of the first AIDS patients and the dismay they provoked in doctors powerless to help them. As David Ho, a physician at the Cedars-Sinai Medical Center, recalled, those early patients "looked like concentration camp survivors." Adding to the dismay was the fact that the causes were "completely unknown." As the true extent of the epidemic became evident—in 1982 the number of AIDS cases in the United States totaled 593; two years later there were nearly 7,000 cases and there had been over 4,000 deaths—AIDS came to be regarded as a plague (the "gay plague" to be specific) and the signal of a disastrous return to a former historical epoch when *the* plague and other epidemic diseases had routinely ravaged human communities. If Legionnaires' disease had been a warning to an overly complacent public health profession, then AIDS was the epidemic that drove home the lesson: despite vaccines, antibiotics, and other medical technologies, infectious disease had not been banished but posed a continuing and present threat to technologically advanced societies. Worse, as scientists learned more about the disease and its origins, it soon became apparent that sex and medical technologies—in particular, the wide provision of hypodermic needles and reusable syringes via public health programs and other humanitarian medical initiatives in Africa, plus blood banks and blood transfusion services—had greatly amplified transmission of the virus, transforming what had been scattered, isolated cases in Africa into a widely dispersed infection which eventually became a pandemic. Even so, no one could have imagined that by the end of the twentieth century 14 million people would have died of AIDS globally and 33 million more would be living with the virus. Or that by 2015, a further 36 million people around the world would have contracted HIV, and some 40 million would be dead, a figure that approaches the mortality of the Spanish flu.

As we shall see, the AIDS pandemic was not only the result of technological interventions; as with psittacosis, economic, social, and cultural factors also likely played a part. In particular, the emergence of AIDS appears to have been connected to the construction in the colonial period of new railways and roads in equatorial regions of Central Africa, projects that fueled the influx of male laborers into rural areas, destabilizing gender relations and fostering a culture of prostitution in Léopoldville (Kinshasa) and other large towns and cities. The loosening of sexual taboos following gay liberation was a similarly important factor in the spread of AIDS in the United States, particularly in cities like New York and San Francisco where bathhouses became venues for unprotected anal sex between men boasting multiple sexual partners. However, it would appear that such practices only contributed to the explosion of AIDS in America *after* HIV had been imported to the United States from Haiti in the late 1960s.

In many respects, AIDS is the exception to the epidemics and pandemics canvassed in this book. Unlike influenza or Legionnaires' disease, medical researchers could hardly be accused of being blinded by overconfidence in 1981. Nor could the CDC be accused of being complacent about the threat posed by sexually transmitted diseases in the early 1980s, or of failing to recognize AIDS's peculiar constellation of symptoms sooner. On the contrary, AIDS might have continued its slow, stealth-like spread for several more years had it not been for key conceptual advances in oncology and new laboratory technologies that, for the first time, gave clinicians the possibility of identifying the depletion of CD4 cells that is the signature of advanced HIV infection, and medical researchers the ability to continuously grow T cells in culture. Indeed, reflecting on the history of AIDS, Robert Gallo, the NIH cancer specialist who would share credit for the discovery of HIV with Luc Montagnier of the Pasteur Institute, argued that had AIDS struck in 1955, scientists would have been "in a dark box," so limited was the contemporary understanding of retroviruses and scientists' ability to study them. "No one would have believed in this kind of virus. They did not even know what this kind of virus was," he told an interviewer in 1994. Even in the 1960s and early 1970s, he argued, scientists would have struggled to comprehend HIV. Or, to put it another way, the AIDS epidemic broke out at precisely the moment when, for the first time in history, scientists working in oncology and the specialized area of human retrovirology were inclined to believe that a retrovirus might be the cause of the peculiar new syndrome and possessed the tools and technology to test the hypothesis. Even so, from the beginning of the hunt for the virus of AIDS, research was clouded by presumptions about what sort of retrovirus HIV would turn out to be, and nowhere more so than in the mind of Gallo.

TODAY, IN AN ERA of antiretroviral drugs, when a diagnosis of AIDS is no longer an automatic death sentence, it is easy to forget the panic, hysteria, and stigma of the early days of the pandemic. For conservative politicians such as Jesse Helms, the former Republican senator from North Carolina, and Moral Majority leader Jerry Falwell, AIDS was nothing less than "God's judgment" and divine retribution for homosexuals' "perverted" lifestyles. Others argued that the virus had something to do with voodoo; hence, the way it appeared to target Haitians. Still others thought it had been transported to Earth on the tail of a comet from outer space, or that the virus had been incubated in a bioweapons lab by the CIA with the connivance of the Pentagon and Big Pharma.

In fact, HIV is a special type of virus called a retrovirus. Due to its long latency and gradual onset, it is also classed as a lentivirus (from the Latin term for slow). When a person is first infected with HIV, the immune system produces antibodies to fight off the virus. This process of acute infection can take anywhere from two weeks to three months. During this period, virus levels in the blood are very high and patients are extremely infectious. Victims may also experience flu-like symptoms such as fever, rash, muscle aches, and joint pains, but frequently the symptoms are so mild they pass unnoticed. After seroconversion, HIV usually betrays no further outward sign of its presence for several years. Instead, it works by stealth, silently parasitizing CD4 cells and colonizing the lymphatic system. During the silent phase of infection, HIV uses the machinery of CD4 cells to make copies of itself and spread throughout the body. At each stage, CD4 cells are repeatedly activated and die off. This cycle of activation followed by cell death continues until the body's capacity for replenishing CD4 cells is exhausted, a process that takes around ten years, but can be shorter or longer. Eventually, without an adequate supply of CD4 cells, the immune system can no longer signal B cells to produce antibodies, or CD8 cells—also known as T cells—to kill infected cells. It is at this point that a victim becomes susceptible to opportunistic infections and develops prominent signs of illness. Until then, however, HIV is quiescent: it lies hidden from view inside CD4 and other immune cells.

Measuring CD4 cells is the most important laboratory indicator of a person's immune status and how well their immune system is coping with the virus. Viral load shows the amount of virus in the blood and gives an indication of the risk of progression and transmission, but without the ability to count Michael's CD4 cells, Gottlieb would have had no idea that his immune system was compromised and that he might be the victim of a new condition. In retrospect, it is astonishing to think that this technology became available at precisely the moment when AIDS first emerged in Los Angeles and other US cities. That the technology was available at UCLA and other hospital immunology departments could largely be attributed to the work of an Argentine émigré, César Millstein, and a German biologist, Georges Köhler. In 1975, these scientists found a way to produce an immortal cell line capable of producing endless quantities of antibodies that targeted specific antigens. Known as monoclonal antibodies—or Mabs for short—the technology removed the need to laboriously isolate and purify antibodies from laboratory cultures, and was soon being used in everything from the rapid typing of blood and tissue, to the development of new drugs against infectious diseases. Soon, Mabs were also aiding the study of leukemia, and by 1981 commercial Mab technologies also became available to distinguish one population of T cells from another. Thus it was that in the winter of 1981 Gottlieb's colleague found a virtual absence of CD4 cells in Michael's blood, suggesting that his symptoms were the result of an immune deficiency.

If it is impossible to imagine AIDS being diagnosed without new Mabs technologies, it is also inconceivable that the virus would have been isolated without conceptual advances in oncology and knowledge of lentiviruses. The first lentivirus was described in 1954 by an Icelandic researcher investigating an outbreak of visna, a slow disease of sheep characterized by pneumonia and brain plaques similar to the demyelination of the central nervous system seen in multiple sclerosis. This was followed, three years later, by the description of kuru among members of the Fore tribe of Papua New Guinea highlands. A neurodegenerative disorder, kuru produces a steady deterioration of brain tissue similar to Bovine Spongiform Encephalopathy (BSE), also known as "mad cow disease." Like BSE, kuru is thought to be due to the transmission of an infectious protein called a prion. The difference is that whereas BSE is caused by eating food contaminated with prions from the brains and spinal cords of infected cattle, kuru most likely resulted from funerary cannibalism practices in which the Fore consumed the brains of dead relatives.

In parallel with discoveries of new lentiviruses, in the 1950s scientists were also describing new oncoviruses.* These viruses included mouse leukemia and Burkitt's lymphoma, a rare jaw tumor especially prevalent in children in Uganda and other parts of East Africa with high rates of malaria, which was later found to be due to the Epstein-Barr virus, a close cousin of herpes. Until the 1960s, it was thought that all viruses, including oncoviruses, replicated by inserting their DNA into animal cells and co-opting the cell's machinery to make multiple copies. The only difference in the case of oncoviruses was that, instead of being lytic and killing infected cells, they entered into a state of symbiosis with cells and caused them to replicate. However, this theory hit a major roadblock with the finding that the oncovirus of feline leukemia contained the "messenger" molecule, ribonucleic acid (RNA), rather than DNA, thereby violating one of the central tenets of molecular biology: namely, that genetic information flows from DNA to RNA to protein, not in the opposite direction.

The first breakthrough came with the demonstration in 1970 by David Baltimore of the Massachusetts Institute of Technology and Howard Temin of the University of Wisconsin that certain RNA viruses could achieve integration into cellular genomes with the help

---

*. Oncovirus is the term for any virus that causes cancers or tumors.

of an enzyme, reverse transcriptase. This was an enzyme that they alone, among all RNA viruses, carried, and which enabled them to form DNA from the genes of viral RNA. At first, Baltimore and Temin's discovery of reverse transcriptase was regarded as "heresy," but it was eventually accepted and led to them being awarded the Nobel Prize in 1975. It also led to the coining of the term retroviruses for viruses that possessed this special ability, removing an epistemological obstacle to the understanding of how viral genes could cause cancerous transformations of cells. When a retrovirus infects a cell, the reverse transcriptase takes the clockwise RNA helix and retranscribes it in the reverse direction, rendering it into double-stranded DNA. This DNA "provirus" is then inserted into the host chromosomal DNA with the help of another viral enzyme, integrase. Because the integration site of the provirus is random, it frequently triggers disruptions of adjacent genes, causing cancer. At the same time, integrated into the cell, the virus is protected from attack by the immune system and is effectively invisible to detection with scientific instruments. The virus remains there for the life of the cell, being replicated along with cellular DNA and passed on to daughter cells.

In 1975 only retroviruses causing cancer in animals were known (the classic examples being chicken sarcoma and feline leukemia) and many cancer researchers, discouraged by the contamination of cell lines with infectious viruses of other species, had given up hope of ever finding a human oncogenic retrovirus. Robert Gallo, an ambitious young researcher at the National Cancer Institute, a branch of the NIH, in Bethesda, Maryland, thought otherwise. The son of a metallurgist from Waterbury, Connecticut, with unkempt crinkly hair that betrayed his Italian heritage, Gallo understood right away that reverse transcriptase could add an important dimension to cancer research. He began searching for the enzyme in white blood cells from human leukemia patients. Gallo had two things going for him: a fierce competitive streak—he made no secret of the fact that he hankered after

the Nobel Prize—and a novel technology that enabled him to continuously grow T cells in culture—the T cell growth factor, interleukin-2.
Prior to the late 1970s, oncologists investigating leukemia had to laboriously culture malignant white blood cells on agar media in order to
produce sufficient numbers for the detection of reverse transcriptase.
However, the leukemia cells frequently refused to cooperate, resulting
in frustration and wasted effort. But in 1976 all that changed when
two of Gallo's colleagues at his Laboratory of Tumor and Cell Biology
discovered that a plant derivative stimulated certain T-lymphocytes
and caused them to release a growth factor. This was interleukin-
2, and soon Gallo's lab had demonstrated that it could be used to
prompt leukemia cells to grow and multiply, thereby perpetuating cell
lines indefinitely. Nevertheless, even with this method it took nearly
three years of trial and error before Gallo's group hit paydirt, detect-
ing reverse transcriptase in 1979 in the lymphocytes of a 28-year-old
African American man from Alabama who had been diagnosed with
mycosis fungoides, a type of T-cell lymphoma. Soon after, both Gallo's
laboratory and a group of Japanese researchers found the same virus
in other patients with leukemia and in 1980 named it HTLV, short
for Human T-cell Leukemia Virus. This discovery made headlines
around the world, earning Gallo the prestigious Lasker Prize, and was
followed, in 1982, by the isolation of a second human retrovirus in the
same family, designated HTLV-II by Gallo.

In his book on the discovery of AIDS, *Virus Hunting: AIDS, Cancer
& The Human Retrovirus*, Gallo acknowledges that his interest in HTLV
was partly inspired by the finding, a decade earlier, that the feline leukemia virus more often caused an AIDS-like immune deficiency in
cats than it did leukemia. He was also inspired by research by his Harvard colleague, Myron "Max" Essex, that Japanese infectious disease
wards were full of people who had tested positive for HTLV-I. Nevertheless, there is no doubt that the discovery of HTLV-I paved the way
for the isolation in 1983 at the Pasteur Institute in Paris of the lymph-

adenopathy associated virus (LAV), the virus now known as HIV, by the French researchers Françoise Barré-Sinoussi and Luc Montagnier.

HTLV infects CD4 cells and spreads by blood and sexual contact, often producing leukemias several decades after the originating infection. The difference is that HTLV is oncogenic; for reasons which are not fully understood but which involve a protein called Tax, it causes cells to replicate rather than killing them. However, similar techniques are required to grow the virus continuously in cell cultures, and had Gallo not demonstrated that HTLV depended on reverse transcriptase and was associated with a depletion of CD4 cells, it is unlikely that Barré-Sinoussi and Montagnier would have thought that the retrovirus they were studying might possess similar properties. However, it is also clear that Gallo's conviction that the virus of AIDS was an oncogenic virus, similar to the feline leukemia virus, blinded him to other research avenues that might have seen him isolate HIV before the French. Instead, in May 1983, in a note published in the *Morbidity and Mortality Weekly Report* and followed by a series of articles in *Science*, Gallo announced that a variant of HTLV-I, or its near relative HTLV-II, was most likely the pathogen of AIDS. Unfortunately for Gallo, in the same issue of *Science*, Barré-Sinoussi and Montagnier announced their discovery of LAV. As the virus showed little or weak cross-reactivity with HTLV-I, it was clear that theirs was a different virus. Despite this, at the request of the editors, Montagnier agreed to an abstract, written by Gallo, stating that the French had discovered "a retrovirus belonging to the same family of recently discovered human T-cell leukemia viruses (HTLV), but clearly distinct from each previous isolate." That sentence would leave the Pasteur Institute researchers with a nasty aftertaste, one that would provoke a bitter international dispute over the correct nomenclature of the virus and who had discovered it—a dispute that in turn would engender misunderstandings about HIV's identity and its precise relationship to AIDS, fueling conspiracy theories that persist to this day.

The dispute between Gallo and Montagnier, and the scientific and commercial stakes that lay behind it (one of the fiercest issues was who should collect royalties for the development of an HIV diagnostic test), has been the subject of books by both of the principals and has also been analyzed extensively by other writers. The bad feeling between the French and American scientists was exacerbated by an ill-considered press conference in April 1984 at the US Department of Health and Human Services at which Gallo announced that he had isolated the virus of AIDS and followed up that announcement with four further papers in *Science* in which he named the virus HTLV-III.* In 1986, the dispute appeared to have been settled when the International Committee on the Taxonomy of Viruses renamed the virus HIV and, soon afterwards, Ronald Reagan and Frédéric Mitterrand, who was then the president of France, announced that both groups of scientists deserved equal credit for the discovery, only for the dispute to be reopened in 1990 by new genetic tests suggesting, wrongly as it turned out, that Gallo had misappropriated samples forwarded to his laboratory from the Pasteur Institute in 1983. This is not the time or place to revisit that fraught history or whether in naming the virus HTLV-III Gallo intended to suggest it was related to other viruses in the HTLV family or even that it was the cause of AIDS (he would subsequently say he had never made this claim). However, it is worth dwelling on one aspect of the dispute because it goes to the heart of the question as to what both groups of scientists knew, or thought they knew, about the virus at the time they first posited its etiological role in AIDS, and the extent to which Gallo was blinded by his belief that the AIDS virus belonged to the cancer family of retroviruses.

In the second set of papers published in *Science*, Gallo described how he had isolated HTLV-III from forty-eight patients and spelled

---

* It subsequently emerged that HTLV-III was identical to LAV and was almost certainly a contaminant from a virus that Montagnier had shared with Gallo's lab.

out how to grow the virus continually in laboratory cultures. This was a critical feat. HIV routinely kills the cells it infects, making it difficult to grow the virus in the quantities needed to study its properties and develop a blood test, let alone a vaccine. Indeed, using the new cell line, Gallo's group was already well on the way to developing a prototype screening test (or ELISA), as well as a confirmatory test (known as the "Western blot"). However, in his earlier 1983 paper Gallo had made no mention of the virus's cell-destroying properties, merely observing that it could be immunosuppressive in vitro: that is, it could harm the function of T cells in laboratory cultures. This left open the question of how precisely HTLV, a virus that was known to cause lymphocytes to divide, also resulted in them becoming depleted.

By contrast, the French started from the premise that because the virus reduced and destroyed the numbers of circulating T cells, it would be difficult to isolate in peripheral blood. At this stage, Montagnier's group accepted that it was most likely a retrovirus closely related to, or identical to, HTLV. However, rather than look for it in blood they decided to look for it in fluid taken from the lymph nodes of a presumed AIDS patient, reasoning that there might be higher levels of the virus present in people who were at an earlier stage of illness before most of their T cells had been killed off. Thus it was that on January 3, 1983, a researcher at the Pitié-Salpêtrière Hospital in Paris removed a lymph node from the neck of a 33-year-old man with "lymphadenopathy syndrome"—a condition of chronically swollen lymph glands increasingly prevalent in gay men—and added interleukin-2 to encourage cell-line growth.[*] If the virus had been a species of HTLV, the addition of interleukin-2 should have maintained the culture and its population of T cells, but that is not what hap-

---

[*] The patient was identified in Montangier's laboratory notes by the first three letters of his name, BRU. He was later named by newspapers as Frédéric Brugière, a homosexual who had allegedly had relations with fifty partners a year and who had visited New York City in 1979.

pened. Instead, no sooner had Barré-Sinoussi observed the production of reverse transcriptase by the cultured lymphocytes on January 25, than production of the enzyme reached a peak, before falling back. The virus seemed to be killing the T cells rather than causing them to replicate. Fearing that without a new supply of lymphocytes she would lose the virus, she asked a member of the team to obtain fresh blood from a nearby blood bank. Adding the new source of lymphocytes to the culture, she saw that cell death correlated once again with the detection of reverse transcriptase activity. It was as if the addition of the plasma containing fresh lymphocytes caused the elusive virus to begin gobbling up T cells again, leaving an unmistakable trail of reverse transcriptase, much as a shark leaves a blood trail after attacking its prey. It was at that moment that Barré-Sinoussi realized the virus was killing the T cells, that it was a new retrovirus and that it was almost certainly not Gallo's HTLV. As she later recalled: "It was very easy. We received the first sample at the beginning of 1983 and, fifteen days later, we had the first sign of the virus in the culture."

If Barré-Sinoussi thought the wider world would immediately grasp the significance of her experiment she was wrong, however. The publication of her paper on LAV in the May 1983 edition of *Science* was completely overshadowed by the papers by Gallo and Essex. Not only that, but when in the fall of 1983 Montagnier traveled to an international virology conference held each September in Cold Spring Harbor, New York, and reported finding LAV in about 60 percent of patients with lymphadenopathy syndrome and 20 percent of those with AIDS, and that none of these patients appeared to be infected with HTLV, his findings were fiercely disputed by Gallo. In his book, Gallo would later write of his "regret" about his aggressive questioning of Montagnier and acknowledge his failure to spot LAV's cell-killing properties earlier—a failure that he attributed to the "distortion" of his laboratory's measurement of reverse transcriptase activity due to the fact that tests usually began later in the course of infection, by which

time most of the T cells were already damaged or dying, as well as by
inconclusive immunofluorescent assays that were sometimes positive
for HTLV-I and sometimes not (perhaps because some of the subjects
were infected with both HIV and HTLV simultaneously, or one or
other of the viruses separately). However, in his account of his own
investigation Montagnier argues persuasively that, with the superior
financial resources available to the Americans, had Gallo believed in
the French virus from the very beginning, he "would have rapidly
left us far behind." That is a conclusion with which Gallo reluctantly
concurred, acknowledging that his "overconfidence" that AIDS could
not be a type of retrovirus different from HTLV probably cost him six
months and that he should have solved the problem before Montagnier's group embarked on their first experiment. "AIDS being identified
right after the discovery of the first and second human retroviruses . . .
misled me," Gallo admitted. "As well as leading me right, it also led
me wrong." Or as the historian of science Mirko Grmek put it rather
more directly, "If Gallo had not discovered HTLV-I, he might well have
been the discoverer of HIV."

⤛⤜

IN HER BOOK *Illness as Metaphor*, the cultural critic Susan Sontag
draws attention to the way in which any disease whose causality is
murky and for which treatment is ineffectual tends to be awash with
significance. "First, the subjects of deepest dread (corruption, decay,
pollution, anomie, weakness) are identified with the disease. The disease itself becomes a metaphor. Then, in the name of the disease (that
is, using it as a metaphor), that horror is imposed on other things."
Those words were written in 1978 and were originally inspired by
Sontag's experiences as a cancer patient, when she had been made
to feel that the disease was shameful and somehow her fault, but as
she recognized when she revisited her thesis in the wake of the AIDS
epidemic, her comments applied even more to AIDS. Indeed, by 1989

she argued that the secrecy, shame, and feelings of culpability experienced by cancer patients in the 1970s had to a large extent been replaced by those of AIDS patients. This was particularly the case for homosexual men and other designated at-risk groups, such as intravenous drug users, whose dangerous behaviors were thought to have somehow invited the affliction. Such groups, she argued, had been made to feel like "a community of pariahs." Worse, whereas in the case of cancer, culpability for illness had been linked to unhealthy habits such as cigarette smoking and excessive drinking, the unsafe behavior that produced AIDS was viewed as something more than weakness of will. "It is indulgence, delinquency—addictions to chemicals that are illegal and to sex regarded as deviant." The result was that what should have been considered an individual "calamity" that invited sympathy for the afflicted, was judged harshly "as a disease not only of sexual excess but of perversity," resulting in the widespread stigmatization of people with AIDS.

At what point this stigmatization morphed into hysteria and panic about the threat that such patients posed to wider society is harder to say. Initially, the public responded with indifference to news of the outbreak, perhaps taking their cue from White House press spokesman Larry Speakes who, when asked by a reporter in October 1982 whether the Reagan administration had any reaction to the CDC's announcement of over six hundred cases of the mysterious new disease, famously responded, "I don't know anything about it." This indifference was due partly to ignorance and partly to prejudice about a disease that was thought to affect only homosexuals. As long as AIDS was framed as a disease of gay lifestyles, and therefore not a problem for "straight" society, it could be safely ignored by mainstream politicians. Instead, Ronald Reagan's administration, backed by the Republican-controlled Senate, starved AIDS researchers of funds, forcing scientists at the NIH and CDC to beg and steal money from other programs. Indeed, for the first three years of the epidemic, Reagan refused to mention the "A"-word, only referring to AIDS in public for the first time in the fall of 1985. By then, of course, the actor Rock Hudson had been forced to admit that he had the dreaded disease, issuing a press release from his sickbed at the American Hospital in Paris, and the CDC was reporting that more than 10,000 people had been diagnosed with AIDS, many of them children and hemophiliacs. According to David France, a contributor to the New York *Native* who would go on to make an Oscar-nominated film telling the story of how AIDS activists took on the scientific establishment in the quest for medications that would prolong their lives, Hudson's announcement was a game changer. "We prayed for a day when the disease struck someone who mattered," he wrote. In particular, it prompted reporters to ask embarrassing questions about why the Hollywood icon had been forced to seek treatment in Paris, unleashing a wave of publicity that finally broke the administration's murderous silence around AIDS and persuaded the White House to release much needed funds for research into experimental treatments, such as AZT. What France and other activists did not foresee is that it would also unleash a wave of fear and hysteria.

This hysteria can be traced to three factors: the first was the discovery that AIDS was a blood-borne disease that could also be spread by intravenous drug use and the sharing of needles and that it was in the nation's blood supply; the second was poor public health messaging and the use of vague terms such as "bodily fluids," which gave the impression that you could contract AIDS from saliva and sneezes, or even from touching an object that had been handled by someone with AIDS; and the third was the realization that the disease was due to a deadly new type of virus that might also be capable of heterosexual spread, and there were no drugs available to treat it, making diagnosis equivalent to a death sentence. Suddenly, it seemed, there was no safe ground, no place that was secure from the virus. Instead, AIDS rapidly took on the aspect of a contagion, sparking what the journalist Randy Shilts called an "epidemic of fear."

Looking back, Shilts had little doubt that scientists and medical experts—not the media—were largely responsible for this new framing of AIDS. In March 1983 the CDC had named the principal risk groups as homosexual men with multiple sexual partners, heroin addicts who injected drugs, Haitians, and hemophiliacs—the so-called "four Hs." However, two months later, the *Journal of the American Medical Association* gave a completely different impression, publishing an article about eight cases of unexplained immune deficiency among children in Newark, New Jersey, four of whom had died, and stated that "sexual contact, drug abuse or exposure to blood products is not necessary for disease transmission." Worse, in an accompanying editorial, Anthony Fauci, the head of the NIAID and the leading federal AIDS researcher, compounded the offense by stating there was a "possibility that routine close contact, as within a family household" could spread the disease. In case the press failed to get the message, the American Medical Association also issued a press release headlined, "Evidence Suggests Household Contact May Transmit AIDS," in which it quoted Fauci as saying that the possibility of "non-sexual, non-blood borne transmission" had "enormous implications" and that "If routine close contact can spread the disease, AIDS takes on an entirely new dimension." The release was immediately taken up by Associated Press, who interpreted it to mean that the general population was at greater risk of AIDS than had previously been thought, and flawed versions of the AP story were soon running in *USA Today* and other newspapers. Within days, officials in San Francisco began distributing face masks and rubber gloves to police and fire officers, and an image of an officer trying on one of the masks appeared in several metropolitan dailies, becoming what Shilts calls "a virtual emblem of the AIDS hysteria" sweeping the nation. Not long after, other police departments began agitating for the same masks, and California dentists were advised to take similar precautions.

Although Fauci would subsequently accuse the media of taking his comments out of context and of failing to appreciate the nuances of his editorial, his comments were compounded by the language employed by health officials who, nervous about offending public sensibilities by specifying that AIDS was spread through "semen" and blood, adopted the euphemism "bodily fluids." The result was that it was a year before Fauci corrected the misunderstanding by clarifying in an article for another peer-reviewed journal that there was no evidence that AIDS could be transmitted by routine household or social contact.

The capacity of this new framing of AIDS to provoke panic and hysteria was driven home by the news in July 1985 that a middle school in Kokomo, Indiana, was refusing to readmit a fourteen-year-old hemophiliac, Ryan White, who had been infected with AIDS following a routine blood transfusion a year earlier. Even though White had been declared fit by doctors, the local school corporation had bowed to pressure from hysterical parents worried about their children sharing a classroom with an AIDS "carrier." The hysteria spread rapidly to other school districts, including New York, where, in an article headlined "The New Untouchables," *Time* reported that some nine hundred parents at an elementary school in Queens were refusing to let their children attend classes because of one AIDS-infected second grader. Soon, newspapers in other countries were carrying stories of similarly hysterical overreactions. In England, the *Sun* newspaper reported that AIDS was "spreading like wildfire" and that a victim of the disease had been entombed in concrete in a cemetery in North Yorkshire "as a precaution." In Brussels, according to the *Daily Mirror*, a court had been emptied in seconds after a prisoner declared that he was infected with the virus, prompting the judge, clerks, and several prison officers to flee in terror. Meanwhile, back in the United States, Masters and Johnson warned that AIDS could lurk on toilet seats, while in Chicago a worried motorist who had just run over a gay pedestrian telephoned an AIDS hotline wanting to know whether he should decontaminate his car. Even family physicians, whose Hippocratic oath meant they owed a duty of care to *all* patients, found excuses not to treat people with AIDS or to refer them to specialist colleagues.

In the early months of the epidemic, it was common for both network news anchors and gay men to refer to AIDS as a lifestyle disease associated with homosexuality and living in the "fast lane." In retrospect, it can be seen that this construction was a product of the initial case descriptions used by CDC epidemiologists to identify the main risk groups. Thus in the first report about the new syndrome in the *Morbidity and Mortality Weekly Report,* Curran had floated the hypothesis that the incidence of PCP in Gottlieb's UCLA patients suggested "an association between some aspect of homosexual lifestyle or disease acquired through sexual contact." This was followed in July 1981 by a second report in the same journal, detailing how KS had been diagnosed in twenty-six male patients in New York. Coinciding with an article in the *New York Times,* in which Friedman-Kien, himself a gay man, provided fifteen more cases of KS to a reporter, it was at this point that the wider medical community and the media began to talk about a "rare cancer" and, afterwards, a "gay plague."

Perhaps the CDC's most significant contribution to the stigmatization of homosexuals was the publication in 1982 of a study of patients with KS and other opportunistic infections in Los Angeles and Orange Counties. Known as the Los Angeles cluster study, it was this that introduced the public to perhaps the most notorious patient in the history of infectious disease after Typhoid Mary: French Canadian flight attendant Gaetan Dugas. Subsequently immortalized as "patient zero" by the journalist Randy Shilts in his popular history of AIDS, *And the Band Played On,* Dugas was ready-made for demonization as the epidemic's "bad guy." A complex character who boasted hundreds of casual sexual partners, Dugas refused to give up his addiction to bathhouses even as his body was ravaged by KS and evidence mounted that AIDS might be sexually transmitted. After Dugas's death in March 1984, Friedman-Kien and other physicians were quick to label him a "sociopath." But such judgments tend to ignore the extent to which, in the early years of the epidemic, knowledge about AIDS's etiology and its routes of transmission were uncertain and subject to conjecture. They also obscured the fact that, though skeptical of medical claims about gay lifestyles contributing to the epidemic, Dugas was very helpful to William Darrow, the CDC sociologist who led the study, providing him with the names of 72 of the roughly 750 men he had slept with in the previous three years. Ironically, it was this frankness about his sexual history, and his willingness to assist epidemiologists in reconstructing the pathways of transmission, that would result in Dugas being accorded a starring role in Darrow's study and Shilts's book, leading to what the historian of medicine Richard McKay calls Dugas's "posthumous notoriety."

In contrast to microbiologists and other laboratory-based investigators, epidemiologists tend to privilege multifactorial models of disease: that is, they believe a given disease may have a number of causes or antecedents, a combination of which may be required to produce the disorder. By investigating this "web of causes," the aim is to identify the disorder's most vulnerable point and intervene, thereby curtailing further spread of the pathogen before its identity is known. Prior to the identification of the virus in 1983, this was the situation that confronted Curran and his colleagues in the STD division of the CDC. At that point no one realized that the epidemic was due to a new virus unknown to medical science, let alone that it could be transmitted in blood as well as semen. However, as discussed above, new medical technologies had already made the depletion of CD4 cells visible to medical researchers, alerting physicians and epidemiologists to the immune deficiency that is one of AIDS's hallmarks. Moreover, the CDC had just completed a multiyear, multisite study of hepatitis

B, a disease which is often sexually transmitted and whose prevalence was known to be very high among homosexual men. In analyzing the data, the researchers found that blood markers for the disease were significantly associated with, among other factors, having a large number of male sexual partners and engaging in sexual practices involving anal contact. At the same time, researchers at the NIH and elsewhere were growing concerned about the increase in CMV transmission among homosexuals—a phenomenon that had never been seen on such a scale before among adults, homosexual or otherwise. The analysts who read these studies were mostly heterosexual and middle-aged and had little understanding of gay lifestyles, so it is not surprising that they were quick to link the epidemic in STDs to the gay liberation movement and its attendant world of bathhouses and anonymous hookups. In addition, as Garrett reports, many researchers began to worry that these same gay lifestyles might be altering the "ecology" of STDs. In this way, the same factors that made the new syndrome visible to epidemiologists for the first time also contributed to the stigmatization of gay men and their supposed behaviors, and it was not long before the CDC was referring to the disorder as gay-related immune deficiency (GRID).

This stigmatization of gay men's lifestyles was almost certainly inadvertent. Curran, who headed the CDC's new Task Force on Kaposi's Sarcoma and Opportunistic Infections, had previously worked closely with the gay community to evaluate the hepatitis B vaccine, so he was well aware of the community's sensitivities. However, as an STD specialist he also could not help but favor the sexual transmission theory. This bias deepened when Curran ordered a "quick and dirty" survey of 420 males attending venereal disease clinics in San Francisco, New York, and Atlanta and then selected 35 for interview. Two patterns of behavior caught the task force's attention: first, the men had had many sexual partners in the past year (the median was eighty-seven), and second, they had frequently used marijuana, cocaine, and amyl nitrate poppers. In particular, there was a close association with the number of sexual partners and the use of poppers. This soon led to the suggestion that it might be exposure to amyl nitrate, rather than the sexual behavior of the subjects, which caused the immune deficiency. The theory received a boost with a study showing that exposure to amyl nitrate was associated with an increased risk of KS in New York, and an investigation of eleven immunocompromised men with PCP, also from New York, seven of whom were identified as drug "abusers" (what received rather less attention was the fact that five of the men had described themselves as heterosexual). However, with the publication of the first installment of the Los Angeles cluster study, and even more so with the publication of Darrow's expanded study linking forty homosexual male AIDS patients in ten US cities, this theory gradually gave way to the sexual transmission hypothesis, prompting news networks to talk about the "gay plague." In particular, Darrow reported that the linked men were more likely than nonlinked controls to have met sexual partners in bathhouses and to have participated in "fisting" (manual-rectal intercourse). Darrow also pointed out that the index patient in the cluster study diagram had had approximately 250 different male sexual partners each year from 1979 through 1981, and that eight of his named partners were AIDS patients, four from Southern California and four from New York. Darrow would later claim that the "O" indicating the index patient in the cluster diagram stood for "Out[side]-of California," not zero. However, Shilts reports that when he visited the CDC to speak to members of the task force, officials were already using the term "Patient Zero" and he immediately thought, "Ooh, that's catchy."*

Whether or not Darrow meant to brand Dugas Patient Zero by des-

---

* Patient zero is a trope that crops up time and again in narrative accounts of epidemics. In epidemiological terms, patient zero is simply the index case; but in nonfiction and novelistic accounts, patient zero is the embodiment of the pathogen and the personification of the infection about to burst forth in society.

ignating him the index case, the L.A. Cluster Study gave the impression that this was where AIDS in America had begun. This impression was reinforced by Shilts's unmasking of Dugas and the revelation that the air steward had made frequent trips to France and, perhaps, to Africa, a continent long feared as a seat of plagues. The result was that in the hands of Shilts and other journalists, Dugas rapidly became a "super spreader" and the prime suspect in the mass murder of hundreds of young men. Thus it was that on October 6, 1987, shortly after the publication of *And The Band Played On*, the tabloid *New York Post* published a front-page story with the headline, "The Man Who Gave Us AIDS." Even supposedly serious news outlets embraced Shilts's partial narrative, with CBS's *60 Minutes* describing Dugas as both the "central victim and victimizer" of the epidemic, and the *National Review* dubbing the Canadian flight attendant "the Columbus of AIDS." Perhaps the most shameful moment came at the end of the year when *People* magazine published an article naming Dugas as one of the "25 most intriguing people of '87" and speculating that it was his "fierce sexual drive" that had given impetus to the epidemic. The article prompted one reader to scrawl "Pervert" and an arrow in a red pen next to Dugas's picture and mail the article to the San Francisco AIDS Foundation.

The perception that Dugas was the main culprit for America's AIDS epidemic was only finally debunked in 2016 when scientists examined stored blood taken from gay and bisexual men in the late 1970s in San Francisco and New York City and found that they already carried antibodies to the main pandemic strain of HIV, suggesting that the index case had probably arrived in New York in around 1970. Not only that, but when scientists examined the genetic sequences in detail, they found them to be similar to HIV strains found in the Caribbean, particulary Haiti, but with enough differences to suggest the virus had already been circulating and mutating on both coasts of America since 1970. When scientists compared these with blood taken from Dugas, they found that Dugas's HIV genome fell right in the middle of the phylogenetic tree of these strains, proof not only that Dugas had not introduced HIV to the U.S. but that his sexual activity had not been a significant factor in the spread of AIDS in the United States.

What makes the stigmatization of Dugas all the more unfortunate is that by early 1982 the CDC had good reason to believe that homosexuals were not the only victims of AIDS and that sexual intercourse was not the only means of transmission, but it took them some time to revise their blinkered view. The first clue had come in September 1981 when infectious disease specialists at Miami's Jackson Memorial Hospital noticed similar symptoms in men and women of Haitian origin. The same month, pediatricians in Miami and New York recognized the same syndrome in children born to Haitian mothers, but when they brought the cases to the attention of the CDC, agency officials were reluctant to believe them. However, by the following summer the CDC task force was hearing of more and more cases of PCP in heterosexuals who were injecting drug users, leading them to believe that GRID might also be transmitted intravenously. At around the same time, the CDC received the first reports of severe PCP in hemophiliacs. The cases involved three men from Denver, Colorado and Westchester, New York—parts of the country not yet known to be affected by the epidemic. Ominously, none of the men had a history of homosexuality or needle sharing, but all three had been given multiple injections of Factor VIII, a blood coagulant concentrate pooled from the plasma of thousands of donors across the United States. This was followed, in July 1982, by a report that a disease identical to GRID had broken out among thirty-four Haitian emigrants to the United States, most of them heterosexual men who had arrived in the country in the previous two years. In addition, eleven cases of KS were discovered in the Haitian capital, Port-au-Prince. However, it was only in September 1982, after the agency learned that a pediatrician at the University of California Medical Center was treating an infant with

PCP and that the two-year-old had received multiple blood transfusions at birth, that the CDC finally dropped the term GRID and in September 1982 began referring to the disease as AIDS.

BY THE LATE 1980S, with half of America's hemophiliacs infected with HIV—70 percent in the case of those with the most severe form of the disorder—few experts doubted that AIDS was also a blood-borne disease. But that still left open the question of where the virus had come from and how it had infected such a diverse range of social and ethnic groups—homosexuals, Haitians, heroin addicts, hemophiliacs— before anyone in the medical community had noticed. By now every region of the world had reported at least one case of HIV, leading the WHO to suggest that the pandemic had emerged simultaneously on three continents. However, few people accepted this theory, not least because it was in Africa that AIDS appeared to be spreading most quickly. Moreover, by the close of the decade, tests on historical serum samples had demonstrated that HIV had already been present in Zaire and Uganda in the 1970s. That these HIV-infected patients included women and children suggested that HIV might have been seeded in heterosexual populations in Central Africa several decades before it arrived in America. Coupled with the growing awareness of AIDS infections among Haitians, this suggested an African point of origin.

The first evidence for this hypothesis had come in 1983 when serum collected from a woman in the obstetrics ward of Mama Yemo Hospital in Kinshasa tested positive for LAV. The findings prompted Montagnier to conduct further tests on archived blood samples from Zaire dating back to 1970, many of which also turned out to be positive for the virus. At the same time, using the ELISA test, Gallo began examining stored blood samples that had been collected by the National Cancer Institute in 1972 and 1973 from schoolchildren in Uganda as part of a study of Burkitt's Lymphoma. To his astonishment, these showed that two-thirds of the Ugandan children were infected with HTLV-III.

In 1983 Peter Piot, a Belgian microbiologist who had become concerned about the number of wealthy Zairians presenting with symptoms of immune deficiency at his tropical diseases clinic in Antwerp, decided to investigate the full extent of the problem in Zaire. Focusing on Mama Yemo Hospital, where doctors had first noted AIDS-like wasting symptoms in the late 1970s, he found that during a three-week period scores of patients on the wards were infected with AIDS. Subsequently he was joined by Jonathan Mann, a former CDC epidemiologist who would go on to become director of the WHO Global Program on AIDS, and the pair began gathering further epidemiological data as part of *Project SIDA*, the first and largest AIDS research project in Africa. By 1986, they had established that AIDS was an escalating problem in Zaire and Rwanda, with up to 18 percent of blood donors and pregnant women infected with HIV. They also noted that the syndrome affected men and women more or less equally, and that most of the men surveyed considered themselves heterosexuals. If this was not enough to dispel the canard that AIDS was a predominantly homosexual disease, researchers went on to report that up to 88 percent of commercial sex workers in Kinshasa and the Rwandan capital Kigali were also infected with the virus, with a similarly high frequency of HIV infections in their clients.

However, perhaps the best evidence that the virus had been present in Africa for some time came from retrospective tests of stored serum samples collected during the Ebola outbreak in Yambuku in 1976. Of the 659 samples drawn from patients in villages close to the Catholic mission hospital, 0.8 percent tested positive for HIV. But while the shocking symptoms of Ebola and the high mortality rate had immediately attracted the attention of investigators from the CDC and elsewhere, no one had noticed these HIV infections at the time. If evidence were ever needed of HIV's cunning, this was it. Unlike Ebola, and other animal-origin viruses that are new to humans, HIV does not draw attention to itself by killing its host suddenly or violently. Instead, the virus has evolved a slow-but-sure strategy that enables it to infect human cells and replicate unnoticed. The result is that people parasitized by HIV can live and quietly pass on the virus for ten years or more before showing any signs of illness. Indeed, it was only in 1985–1986 when three of the villagers in Yambuku developed illnesses suggestive of AIDS that scientists thought to screen the local population for HIV. Interestingly, this survey turned up similar levels of HIV infection as a decade earlier, suggesting that, in rural areas of Africa at least, the virus had made little progress in ten years. This would be an important clue to its epidemiology.

As scientists began screening other collections of archived sera, so other missed alarms came to light, this time in Europeans. One of the most interesting was that of the Danish surgeon Grethe Rask, who had died in Copenhagen in 1977, after suffering a range of AIDS-like opportunistic infections, including PCP. At the time she became ill, in 1974, Rask had been working in Kinshasa, but prior to that, between 1972 and 1975, she had been based in Abumonbazi, a rural hospital sixty miles north of Yambuku. Initial tests in 1985 using an early version of ELISA were negative for HIV, but when the tests were repeated two years later with more sophisticated assays they were positive for the virus. Another case was that of a Norwegian family— father, mother and nine-year-old daughter—all of whom had died of AIDS-like symptoms in 1976. In 1988, retrospective tests showed they all had HIV, and since the daughter had been born in 1967, this suggested the mother had already been infected by that date. Intriguingly, the father had been a sailor who had visited a number of ports in West Africa in the early 1960s, including Nigeria and Cameroon in 1961–1962. The hypothesis was that at one of these ports he may have slept with a prostitute and contracted the virus.

By the mid-1980s, evidence of similarly early cases of AIDS were also coming to light in Africa. The first HIV-positive specimen was isolated from a Bantu man who had given blood in 1959 in Léopoldville, the old Belgian colonial name for Kinshasa. The blood specimen had lain in a refrigerator for twenty-seven years. At the time, it was not possible to identify to which HIV group the specimen belonged, but in the 1990s it became possible to amplify genetic material using a new technique called polymerase chain reaction (PCR), and in 1998 scientists established that it belonged to the same group responsible for the vast majority of pandemic infections. Then, in 2008, a group of scientists writing in *Nature* announced they had sequenced HIV from another specimen, also from Léopoldville. This specimen had been taken from the lymph gland of a woman in 1960, after which it had been stored in the pathology department of the University of Kinshasa. Although the material was badly fragmented, using PCR the team, led by Michael Worobey, an evolutionary biologist at the University of Arizona, were able to sequence a few strands of DNA and RNA. After amplifying the genetic material, Worobey then compared the virus to the earlier isolate from Léopoldville and established that it was a closely related subtype. The next stage was to use a molecular clock to calculate how long it would have taken the two viruses to have diverged from one another. This produced a date for the common ancestor virus between 1908 and 1933 (with a median of 1921). Given the uncertainty of molecular clock calculations (RNA does not mutate at the same rate as DNA), these measures should be viewed with a degree of skepticism. However, there is little doubt that HIV was present in Léopoldville by 1959, and, if Worobey's calculations are correct, very possibly as early as 1921.

Using the same PCR techniques, scientists have also gone on to study current circulating strains of HIV. To date, these studies have shown that there are two main types of HIV: HIV-1, which is highly transmissible and is responsible for the vast majority of infections worldwide, and HIV-2, which circulates mainly in West Africa and is associated with comparatively low levels of virus in the blood. To complicate the picture further, HIV-1 has been divided into four groups and one of these groups, group M, has been subdivided into ten subtypes. In addition, if individuals are infected with more than one subtype, the subtypes can swap genes and form new recombinant strains. The result is an alphabet soup highly confusing to the layman.

Nevertheless, today few scientists doubt that AIDS originated in Africa. This is not only because the two oldest isolates of HIV come from Kinshasa, but because nowhere else in the world does the virus show such diversity. HIV evolves only in one direction, from a single model of a virus to an increasingly complex differentiation into subtypes and recombinants, so viral diversity is strong evidence of point of origin. So far, so uncontroversial. But almost everything else about the origins of HIV and its association with AIDS has been contested. For instance, some retrovirus experts, such as Peter Duesberg, a biologist at the University of California, continue to deny that HIV is the cause of AIDS, even though the virus's etiological role has long been accepted by all competent scientific authorities. Similarly, the British writer and journalist Edward Hooper maintains that AIDS can be traced to mass polio vaccination campaigns conducted in Central Africa in the late 1950s (Hooper argues that the inhabitants of the Belgian Congo, Rwanda, and Burundi were given an oral polio vaccine, known as CHAT, contaminated with a simian immune-deficiency virus as a result of the chimpanzee cells used in the production of the vaccine). Hooper's thesis is described in exhaustive detail in his 1999 book, *The River: A Journey Back to the Source of HIV and AIDS*, and on his website, where he continues to wage an increasingly lonely campaign against his scientific critics, the vast majority of whom consider the weight of evidence against his theory overwhelming. Whether or not Hooper or his critics will ultimately be proved right, one of the consequences of his and Duesberg's critiques has been to fuel conspiracy theories about the role of medical science in spreading AIDS and to undermine faith in AZT and other potentially life-saving drug treatments. This is particularly true of South Africa where Thabo Mbeki, who was president from 1999 to 2008 and who had taken advice from Duesberg, refused people access to antiretroviral drugs, thereby resulting in 330,000 unnecessary deaths from AIDS between 2000 and 2005, according to one study. Similarly, there is evidence that Hooper's vaccine contamination theory may have contributed to the distrust of modern polio vaccines, particularly in countries such as Nigeria, Afghanistan, and Pakistan where suspicions about the vaccines and the motivations of international health workers have fueled resistance to mass immunization campaigns, jeopardizing the WHO's attempts to eradicate the disease from its last endemic centers.

Regardless of the truth or otherwise of these theories, no one disputes that both HIV-1 and HIV-2 are descended from simian immunedeficiency viruses (SIVs) that parasitize, respectively, chimpanzees and sootey mangabeys indigenous to Central and West Africa, and which cause simian versions of AIDS. The question is, how did these viruses jump species or "spill over" from monkeys and become widely amplified in human populations?

A leading spillover mechanism is thought to be the hunting and butchering of monkeys captured in the tropical rain forests of Cameroon, Gabon, and the Congo—the region that is home to *Pan troglodytes troglodytes* chimpanzees. When hunters are cut or bitten in the course of capturing the monkeys or when the animals are butchered for the table, their viruses can readily be transferred to humans. Both simian foamy virus (SFV) and the Ebola and Marburg viruses have been acquired from monkeys in this way. Serological tests of pygmies and Bantu huntsmen show that many carry antibodies to SIVs, suggesting that exposure is a common occurrence in nature. Furthermore, from analysis of the genomes of HIV-1 and HIV-2, as well as their various groups and subtypes, it is known that modern HIV viruses are more closely related to their nearest ancestral SIVs than they are to one another. This is evidence that the simian progenitors of human HIVs must have jumped to humans several times in the course of their evolution. However, as only one group of HIV-1—the M group—is responsible for 99 percent of HIV-1 infections worldwide, this also suggests that the AIDS pandemic started not because a lot of people were infected directly from chimpanzees, but because a rare case of infection managed to spread and multiply in humans, something that all the other simian-origin infections that came before and after it had not managed to do. Fortunately, as the isolate taken from the Bantu man in Léopoldville in 1959 belongs to the HIV-1 M group, and it is there that the virus shows the greatest genetic diversity, when and where this event occurred is no longer a matter of conjecture. The pandemic strain of HIV must have been up and running in 1959 in Léopoldville or else in a nearby town in the Belgian or French Congo. It is in answering the question of how this happened that the debate gets interesting.

Broadly speaking, there are two schools of ecological thought. The first is that a combination of bushmeat hunting and economic and social changes driven by colonialism, plus globalization—better road, rail, and plane connections—are sufficient to account for the amplification of the HIV-1 M group in Africa and the subsequent international spread of the virus. The second is that, yes, all those factors are significant but insufficient to explain how this particular group came to be so widely dispersed, first in urban African populations, and later in rural Africa and the rest of the world. This is because, in practice, it is very difficult for a simian virus to establish itself in a new human host. Indeed, many SIVs that cause infection in the short term are rapidly eliminated by the host's immune response. Even if an infection establishes itself in one person, the virus may not spread easily to others. To explain that we need an additional amplifying effect, and the best candidate is provided by medicine. In particular, Jacques Pepin, the leading proponent of this school, points to the reuse of inadequately sterilized hypodermic needles and syringes in the administration of drugs against venereal diseases such as syphilis and tropical diseases such as malaria and yaws in clinics across Africa. As transmission of HIV-1 is ten times more effective through shared needles and syringes than via sexual intercourse, Pepin, a Canadian infectious disease specialist and epidemiologist with broad African experience, argues that these well-meaning medical interventions, many of which were launched during the colonial era, could have given the virus the boost it needed to go from a localized urban epidemic in Léopoldville/Kinshasa to one capable of infecting people as far away as Haiti, New York, and San Francisco.

Unfortunately, it is not possible to go back in time and test Pepin's theory by conducting serological tests of patients who attended clinics in the Congo and elsewhere in the colonial period. The only evidence available is historical serum samples containing surviving fragments of HIV, and inferences from analogous examples of the inadvertent transmission of other blood-borne viruses via needles and syringes used in humanitarian medical programs. A good example of the latter is the tragedy that occurred in Egypt during the government campaigns against schistosomiasis, a potentially fatal disease caused by a parasitic blood fluke spread by snails that live in irrigation channels along the River Nile and other watercourses. Between 1964 and 1982, more than two million injections of tartar emetic were administered each year to 250,000 Egyptians to combat schistosomiasis. On average patients received ten to twelve weekly IV injections with hastily sterilized syringes and needles. The result was a huge increase in hepatitis C, with half of the individuals aged forty and over testing positive for the virus in areas where the schistosomiasis treatment was administered. Similar iatrogenic transmission of hepatitis B occurred in the 1950s during the administration of IV drug treatments for syphilis and gonorrhea at STD clinics in Léopoldville. Of course, while such studies may lend support to Pepin's theory, the evidence, such as it is, must be considered circumstantial and speculative. Like a jury presented with a murderer but no clear-cut murder weapon, we must weigh the evidence and decide who—or, in this case, what—is the most likely culprit.

The first question a jury must address is why, given the fact that humans living in Cameroon, Gabon, Guinea, and Congo-Brazzaville have been in contact with chimpanzees infected with the SIV progenitor of HIV-1 for at least 2,000 years, an epidemic of HIV did not occur sooner? One answer is that in the precolonial period the lack of firearms made it more difficult to hunt apes and the dearth of roads through densely forested areas of Central Africa would have reduced interactions between humans and chimps. Even if, as seems likely, a bushmeat hunter was occasionally infected with HIV and managed to transmit the virus to his wife—or conversely, a cook infected her husband—the worst that might happen is that both would die of AIDS ten years later. Even if the couple were not monogamous, it is highly unlikely that in a remote village setting the virus would have spread far beyond the immediate community. Thus, in the precolonial period such infections would have represented epidemiological dead ends for the virus. However, around the turn of the nineteenth century, these epidemiological conditions began to change, creating new opportunities for progenitor HIV viruses to passage between people and be amplified more widely. The first development was the inauguration in 1892 of a steamship service from Léopoldville to Stanleyville (Kisangani) in the heart of the Congo. By connecting populations that had previously been largely separated, the service created the potential for viruses that might have died out in isolated, rural populations to reach growing urban centers. The population of Léopoldville received another boost in 1898 with the opening of the Matadi-Leo railway, prompting an influx of economic migrants and Belgian administrators. The result was that by 1923 Léopoldville had become the capital of the Belgian Congo. At around the same time, the city began hosting domestic flights and in 1936 inaugurated a direct international service to Brussels. More significant perhaps was the construction of new roads and railways by the French, including the 511-kilometer Chemin de Fer Congo-Ocean railroad. Connecting Brazzaville, on the opposite bank of the Congo River from Léopoldville, with Pointe-Noire on the coast, the railroad required the conscription of some 127,000 male laborers, resulting in the influx in the 1920s and 1930s of adult men into precisely the rural areas that were home to the chimpanzees that carried the progenitor of HIV-1. It also resulted in a constant passage of Africans and Europeans to and from Brazzaville, the new capital of the French federation.

Once these rural-urban connections were up and running, it would not have taken very much to initiate a chain of sexual transmission in Brazzaville or Léopoldville. Pepin argues that one of the most important factors would have been the disruption of social relations that occurred during the colonial period. In particular, he points to the gender imbalances caused by the Belgian policy of conscripting large numbers of men into the labor force while discouraging their wives and families from leaving their villages. This was nowhere more pronounced than in Léopoldville, where by the 1920s men outnumbered women by 4 to 1—an imbalance that encouraged unmarried, working women known as *"femme libres"* to turn to part-time prostitution to supplement their income. Perhaps a bushmeat hunter traveled to Léopoldville and slept with one of these free women. Or perhaps a laborer on the railway alighted at Brazzaville and then caught a ferry to the opposite bank of the Congo River before making his way to a prostitute in Léopoldville. Or perhaps a migrant worker carried the virus to Brazzaville from higher up the Congo River, via one of its tributaries with Cameroon—the HIV-1 M group is most closely related to an SIV indigenous to chimpanzees from southeastern Cameroon; at the time of writing this is the favored scenario. The virus would have had an